IBS

Also by Barbara B. Bolen, PhD

The Everything® Guide to the Low-FODMAP Diet: A Healthy Plan for Managing IBS and Other Digestive Disorders (with Kathleen Bradley, CPC)

Breaking the Bonds of Irritable Bowel Syndrome: A Psychological Approach to Regaining Control of Your Life

IBS Chat: Real Life Stories and Solutions (with Jeffrey D. Roberts, MSEd)

IBS

365

TIPS FOR LIVING WELL

Barbara B. Bolen, PhD

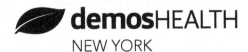

demosHEALTH

NEW YORK

Visit our website at www.demoshealth.com

ISBN: 978-1-936303-86-1
e-book ISBN: 978-1-61705-250-7

Acquisitions Editor: Julia Pastore
Compositor: diacriTech

Medical information provided by Demos Health, in the absence of a visit with a health care professional, must be considered as an educational service only. This book is not designed to replace a physician's independent judgment about the appropriateness or risks of a procedure or therapy for a given patient. Our purpose is to provide you with information that will help you make your own health care decisions.

The information and opinions provided here are believed to be accurate and sound, based on the best judgment available to the authors, editors, and publisher, but readers who fail to consult appropriate health authorities assume the risk of injuries. The publisher is not responsible for errors or omissions. The editors and publisher welcome any reader to report to the publisher any discrepancies or inaccuracies noticed.

Library of Congress Cataloging-in-Publication Data
Bolen, Barbara Bradley.
  IBS : 365 tips for living well / Barbara B. Bolen, PhD.
     pages cm
  Includes bibliographical references and index.
  ISBN 978-1-936303-86-1
  1. Irritable colon—Popular works. 2. Irritable colon—Diet therapy. I. Title. II. Title: Irritable bowel syndrome.
  RC862.I77B66 2015
  616.3'42—dc23
                                2015036142

Special discounts on bulk quantities of Demos Health books are available to corporations, professional associations, pharmaceutical companies, health care organizations, and other qualifying groups. For details, please contact:

Special Sales Department
Demos Medical Publishing, LLC
11 West 42nd Street, 15th Floor
New York, NY 10036
Phone: 800-532-8663 or 212-683-0072
Fax: 212-941-7842
E-mail: specialsales@demosmedical.com

Printed in the United States of America by McNaughton & Gunn.
15 16 17 18 19 / 5 4 3 2 1

This book is dedicated to all of the people who bravely face the challenges of living a life with IBS. This includes those who stumble upon my work during desperate Internet searches, my loyal readers and social media followers, and those who took that big step to prioritize their health and work directly with me. I pledge to continue to walk side by side with you on your journey toward improved digestive health.

Contents

Introduction

As a clinical psychologist, I have helped people with all sorts of life difficulties, most of which my education prepared me to handle. In the early days of my career, one problem kept popping up with my patients—a problem I had never heard of—that of irritable bowel syndrome (IBS). I was shocked by what my patients were telling me—they couldn't work a morning shift, they never went out to dinner, they only wore black pants (!?) and were often in crippling pain. They were frustrated by the fact that their doctors could find nothing wrong with them.

Of course, I wanted to be of help. I was gratified to find that the type of therapy I was trained in—cognitive behavioral therapy (CBT)—had some research support for its effectiveness in reducing these disabling IBS symptoms. I was surprised to see that there was no self-help book that I could recommend to my patients. So I took it upon myself to write one.

Since the publication of my first book, I have continued to learn everything that I can about IBS so as to offer help to those whose lives have been turned upside down by this complicated health problem. Doors have opened to me and I have been blessed to be able to share my knowledge on a worldwide scale. However, IBS is a tricky problem; a comprehensive approach is necessary to bring about symptom relief. It can be challenging to try to put all these pieces together in a way that feels manageable.

IBS: 365 Tips for Living Well is thus offered as a one-stop shop, if you will. The book is filled with easy-to-find nuggets of information, covering every aspect of life with IBS. With this easy-to-dip-into format is that there is no need to be overwhelmed by the amount of information. You can take it in at your own comfortable pace. I trust that this comprehensive guide will serve you well in finding solutions to the challenges that IBS brings into your life.

Understanding What Is and Isn't IBS

It is not an understatement to say that IBS is a confusing disorder. Symptoms wax and wane, often with no rhyme or reason. One person's IBS can be very different from the next. Having a strong understanding of what may be going wrong will help you in your efforts to find your way out of the IBS maze. If you are new to IBS, the following tips will help take the mystery out of the disorder. If you have been dealing with IBS for quite some time, skim through—you may find a tidbit that you were not yet aware of.

What Exactly Is IBS?

1 IBS Is a Gastrointestinal (GI) Disorder That Results in Chronic Intestinal Symptoms

IBS is diagnosed when someone experiences the following symptoms on a repeated basis:

- Abdominal pain
- A marked change in the frequency of bowel movements (diarrhea or constipation)
- A marked change in the appearance of stool
- Intestinal gas and bloating
- Mucus in the stool
- Feeling of incomplete evacuation

2 IBS Often Comes with Some Not-So-Typical Symptoms

Although not required for an IBS diagnosis, people who have IBS frequently report these related symptoms:

- Back pain
- Bad taste in mouth or bad breath
- Clammy, cold, or trembling hands
- Dizziness
- Fatigue
- Frequent urination
- Headache
- Heartburn
- Heart palpitations
- Menstrual cramps
- Muscle aches
- Pain during intercourse
- Nausea
- Sleep difficulties

3 · It Is Not Yet Known Why IBS Patients Also Are at Higher Risk for These Other Symptoms

Researchers have not been able to find a reason why IBS patients experience all sorts of weird symptoms alongside their IBS. It is thought that there may be some underlying biological or psychological factor behind it all. It is also possible that their occurrence has to do with some sort of food sensitivity associated with increased permeability of the intestinal lining (leaky gut syndrome).

4 · Some Symptoms Suggest a Different Diagnosis

The following red-flag symptoms are not typical of IBS. If you are experiencing any of these symptoms you need to tell your doctor immediately.

- Anemia
- Fever
- Rectal bleeding
- Significant, unexplained weight loss
- Vomiting

What's Going Wrong?

5 · IBS Is Considered a *Functional Disorder*

One of the most frustrating aspects of IBS is that people can feel so ill, yet their doctors tell them that nothing shows up on tests. This does not mean that the disorder is all in the head! IBS is considered a *functional disorder*. In other words, there is something wrong with the way the digestive system is functioning. It is diagnosed based on the presence of certain symptoms after other disorders have been ruled out.

6 People with IBS Have Motility Problems

Motility has to do with the strength and speed of the muscles within the intestines. If you have diarrhea-predominant IBS (IBS-D), with repeated bowel movements and stool that gets looser and more watery with each trip to the bathroom, your intestines are moving stool through too quickly. If you have constipation-predominant IBS (IBS-C), with infrequent bowel movements and hard-to-pass stools, your intestines are moving stool too slowly. People who have alternating-type IBS (IBS-A) have no predominant motility symptom as they deal with both constipation and diarrhea on a regular basis.

7 People with IBS Have Visceral Hypersensitivity

Visceral hypersensitivity means that pain receptors within inner organs react to stimulation at a lower level than normal. The fact that people with IBS have visceral hypersensitivity is part of the reason that abdominal pain is a hallmark symptom of IBS.

8 Doctors Don't Know for Sure What Causes IBS

Because there is no visible sign of disease process in people who have IBS, doctors do not have any definitive answers as to why someone would develop the disorder and experience motility and visceral sensitivity problems. Researchers are exploring various angles in trying to understand what causes IBS so as to help develop more effective forms of treatment.

9 Even Though There Are No Signs of Visible Inflammation, It May Still Play a Role

Although by definition, no visible inflammation can be seen in the intestines of people with IBS, researchers are looking into the possibility that microscopic inflammation is contributing to problems with IBS.

10 Communication Dysfunction between the Brain and the Gut May Also Be Playing a Role

As we all know, our digestive systems are very reactive to stress. Because the ability to respond quickly to outer threats was key to our survival as a species, our bodies have developed strong ties among the brain, the nervous system, and the intestines. Researchers are finding differences in how this communication network functions, as well as the chemicals involved, in people with IBS as compared to those who don't have the disorder.

11 Gut Bacteria May Be the Key Players behind IBS

Our intestines are populated by trillions of microorganisms. Researchers are looking into the role that an imbalance in gut bacteria may play in both directly causing IBS symptoms and contributing to problems with inflammation and gut-brain communication.

What If It's Not IBS?

12 Make Sure Your Doctor Rules Out Other Disorders

In order for a confirmed diagnosis to be made, other health problems must be ruled out. The next few tips cover some of the more common health problems that share some of the same symptoms as IBS.

13 Get Tested for Celiac Disease

Celiac disease is an autoimmune disorder in which consumption of foods containing gluten causes damage to the small intestine, thus putting a person at risk for serious health problems. Research has shown that IBS patients are at higher risk for celiac disease.

14 Don't Go Gluten Free Until You Have Completed Celiac Disease Testing

The American College of Gastroenterology recommends that all IBS patients be screened for celiac disease. The initial screening for celiac disease is done through the use of a blood test. You *must* be eating foods containing gluten in the time leading up to the test in order for it to be accurate, so don't go gluten free before being screened.

15 You Can Be Sensitive to Gluten, Even if You Don't Have Celiac Disease

There is a condition known as non-celiac gluten sensitivity (NCGS). In this condition, a person experiences gastrointestinal and other symptoms after eating gluten. Such a sensitivity is identified through the use of an elimination diet. Some researchers think that gluten is not necessarily the problem, but rather that fructans—a type of carbohydrate found in many gluten-containing foods—is behind such symptoms. The role of fructans in contributing to IBS symptoms is a key part of the low-FODMAP diet for IBS. More information about an elimination diet and the low-FODMAP diet can be found in Chapter 7.

16 Inflammatory Bowel Disease (IBD) Shares Many of the Same Symptoms as IBS

The inflammatory bowel diseases, ulcerative colitis and Crohn's disease, also result in symptoms of abdominal pain and changes in bowel movement frequency. However, in IBD there are visible signs of inflammation. If a stool test shows any signs of rectal bleeding, your doctor should recommend a colonoscopy to rule out the presence of IBD.

17 Small Intestinal Bacteria Overgrowth (SIBO) Is Thought to Be Responsible for Symptoms in a Subset of IBS Patients

SIBO is a condition in which excessive amounts of gut bacteria are present in the small intestine. If you typically experience symptoms of intestinal gas and bloating within 90 minutes after eating, you may want to talk to your doctor about being tested for SIBO. This is accomplished through the use of a breath test. SIBO is then treated using a specific type of antibiotic.

18 Colon Cancer Has Some Symptoms That Are Very Different from IBS

The symptoms of IBS can be so severe that it is not uncommon for IBS patients to worry that they actually have cancer. Although colon cancer can cause a change in the frequency of bowel movements and the appearance of stool, it also typically presents with fatigue and unexplained weight loss, as well as blood in the stool—symptoms that are *not* typical of IBS. If you have any of those symptoms, tell your doctor immediately.

19 If You Experience Diarrhea Immediately after Eating You May Suffer from Bile Acid Malabsorption (BAM)

A relatively new area of inquiry into the causes of IBS looks at the role of bile acids in diarrhea-predominant IBS (IBS-D). In this condition, excessive amounts of bile are released into the large intestine, causing watery diarrhea. If your symptoms sound like BAM, bring up the subject with your doctor. He or she may decide to have you try a medication that is designed to treat BAM.

20 If Your Symptoms Are Worse after Eating Dairy Products, Get Tested for Lactose Intolerance

A high percentage of IBS patients are lactose intolerant. This is a condition in which a person lacks sufficient amounts of the digestive enzyme lactase, which is necessary for the digestion of lactose, the main sugar in dairy products. Since the lactose is not digested, it is acted upon by gut bacteria, resulting in symptoms of gas, bloating, and diarrhea. Lactose intolerance is diagnosed through the use of a breath test or an elimination diet.

21 Consider Fructose Malabsorption

Many people with IBS have a fructose malabsorption problem. Similar to people with lactose intolerance, those who have fructose malabsorption experience digestive symptoms of gas, bloating, and diarrhea after eating foods containing fructose. Since the fructose is not absorbed at the level of the small intestine, it makes its way to the large intestine where it is acted upon by the gut bacteria, resulting in symptoms. Fructose malabsorption is also diagnosed through the use of a breath test or elimination diet.

22 Other Food Sensitivities May Be Causing Your Symptoms

Food sensitivities appear to cause IBS symptoms in some people. The most common food sensitivities include eggs, some nuts, shellfish, corn, soy, some meats, and coffee. Such sensitivities are diagnosed through the use of an elimination diet. The low-FODMAP diet theory pinpoints common foods that contain high levels of certain carbohydrates, collectively known as FODMAPs, as contributing to IBS symptoms.

A Successful Relationship with Your Doctor

A strong doctor–patient relationship is important for most health disorders but seems to be even more closely tied to positive treatment outcomes when it comes to IBS. Here are some tips for maximizing your interaction with your doctor so that together you can develop an optimal plan for managing your symptoms.

Who to See?

23 See a Doctor for a Proper Diagnosis

If you are having unusual digestive symptoms, it is essential that you speak with your doctor. It is dangerous to try to self-diagnose, as there are other more serious disorders that share some of the same symptoms as IBS.

24 Start with Your Primary Care Doctor

If you have not yet seen a doctor about your symptoms, it is fine to start with your primary care physician. He or she should give you a complete physical, run some blood tests, and give you a test to make sure there is no blood in your stool. Your doctor can make a diagnosis of IBS based on your symptoms, as long as your blood tests come out fine and your stool test is normal.

25 If Necessary, See a Gastroenterologist

Depending on your age and symptom picture, your primary care physician may recommend that you see a gastroenterologist, a type of doctor that specializes in digestive diseases and disorders. You may also decide to see a gastroenterologist if you do not feel that you are getting adequate symptom relief based on your primary care physician's recommendations.

The Importance of a Symptom Diary

26 Start a Symptom Diary

A symptom diary can be a very helpful way for your doctor to get an idea of the digestive symptoms that you have been dealing with. This doesn't have to be anything elaborate, just a simple chart containing information about when you are likely to experience symptoms and what your symptoms are like.

27 Make Note of the Times of Day When You Experience Symptoms

The first column of your diary should list the date and time when your symptoms occurred. In this column you can also add any relevant information about the situation you were in at the time when you were symptomatic. This will allow both you and your doctor to look for any patterns regarding your symptoms.

28 Make Note of What Foods You Have Eaten

The second column is a place to record your meals and snacks. This will provide information as to whether or not certain foods are playing a role in your symptoms.

29 Make Note of Any Other Factors That Might Have Contributed to Your Symptoms

In the third column, you can add anything else that might be relevant. For example, you might include information about your menstrual cycle, poor sleep, or any psychosocial stress.

30 Describe Your Symptoms Simply

In the last column, you can record your symptoms. Simply make note of any problems with constipation, bouts of diarrhea, stool changes, or pain episodes.

31 Rate the Severity of Your Pain on a 1-To-10 Scale

It is often hard to relate to another person's description of pain. Recording your pain level provides a way for your doctor to get a true understanding of how severely you are suffering.

32 Record Your Symptoms over a Two-Week Period

A two-week period provides a nice snapshot for your doctor as to how often you are experiencing symptoms.

Pre-Appointment Prep

33 Be Prepared before Leaving the House

Doctors are busy people. You will get the most out of your visit if you spend a little time preparing for your visit ahead of time. This will help reduce any anxiety you may be feeling about your symptoms and the appointment, and allow you to make sure that your thoughts are well-organized.

34 Make a List of Questions and Concerns to Bring Along

It can happen to the best of us: when we feel anxious, we have a tendency to become tongue-tied. You can get around this by taking a few moments before your visit to make a list of your most pressing questions and concerns. This will help you make sure that the things you are most worried about are addressed.

35 List Any Concerns about Other Possible Diagnoses

IBS is considered a functional disorder in that no visible disease process can be identified through diagnostic testing. It is very common for people who have IBS to worry that their doctor is missing something more serious. Be sure to talk with your doctor about your concerns, so that your worries don't unnecessarily aggravate your symptoms.

36 List Any Questions about Over-the-Counter (OTC) Remedies

As the medication options for IBS are limited, many people turn to OTCs for relief. Make a list of any products that you are currently taking, or are thinking of taking. Not all OTCs are safe for everyone. Your doctor is in the best position to let you know if an OTC is right for you.

37 List Any Questions as to When You Should Take Medicine

If your doctor has prescribed any medication for you, make sure that you know when to take the medication for maximum benefit. Should the medication be taken regularly or only when needed? Are certain times of day better than others? Should the medication be taken with food?

38 Add Any Concerns about Medication Side Effects

Many people react differently to the same medication. Make a quick list of any side effects that you think you are experiencing as a result of any medication you are taking. This will allow your doctor to make a decision about whether you should continue with the prescribed medication.

39 Don't Forget to Ask Any Questions about Diagnostic Procedures

If your doctor recommends that you undergo diagnostic testing, make sure that you understand fully why the test is being recommended and what you can expect to happen before, during, and after the procedure.

At the Appointment

40 Be Open about Your Symptoms

The visit with your doctor is not the time to be embarrassed or modest. Yes, many of us have been trained not to speak openly about our bowel habits, but doctors are very comfortable discussing all aspects of the human body. The more information you can give your doctor about your symptoms, the better able he or she will be to figure out what is going wrong and what you need in order to feel better.

41 Bring a Trusted Friend or Relative

Okay, maybe you don't want someone else in the room with you when you are telling your doctor about the change in your bowel habits and stool appearance. However, it might be nice to have someone with you after the examination, when your doctor is giving you a diagnosis and talking to you about your treatment options. This can be an anxiety-provoking conversation, so having a second set of ears will help ensure that you take in all that your doctor has to say.

Doctor–Patient Relationship

42 Make Sure You Have a Good Working Relationship with Your Doctor

Regardless of health condition, research has shown that having a good relationship with your doctor can affect your treatment outcome. This seems to be especially true for IBS. Make sure that your doctor is open to working collaboratively with you to come up with a comprehensive symptom management plan.

43 Assess Your Doctor's Attention Span

Does your doctor take the time to listen to what you have to say and address your questions and concerns? Research has shown that IBS patients have better treatment outcomes when they feel that their doctor has listened fully and compassionately to their concerns.

44 Assess Your Doctor's Attitude toward Functional Disorders

Some doctors are dismissive of IBS because they do not view it as serious or life-threatening. You will want to choose a doctor who is attuned to quality-of-life issues. If he or she minimizes your distress, because "you know, it's not cancer," do your best to find another doctor.

45 Keep Your Expectations Reasonable

Since we were young, we have been conditioned to think that doctors can make everything better. All we need is a diagnosis and a prescription and we will feel well again. Unfortunately, for now, this is not the case with IBS. There is, as yet, no "cure." Therefore, it may be that the best your doctor can do is to provide you with support and some symptom management strategies.

Making the Most of Your Medical Care

The more you know about the medical side of IBS, the better you will be able to work with your doctor to devise a helpful symptom management plan. Educating yourself can also help clear away some of the mystery of the medical world and therefore help to reduce your anxiety. The tips in this chapter are all designed to help you to become an empowered, educated patient.

Diagnostic Tests

46 Learn about the Types of Diagnostic Tests

Doctors use a variety of tests to help them determine why a person might be experiencing digestive symptoms. None of the following tests are required for an IBS diagnosis, but based on your symptoms, one or more may be recommended to rule out other disorders.

47 A *Colonoscopy* Allows Your Doctor to Examine the Entire Length of Your Large Intestine

A colonoscopy is recommended for everyone over the age of 50. On the day before the procedure you will be asked to follow a liquid diet and to take laxatives to clear out your colon. During the procedure itself, you will be sedated as your doctor inserts a lighted tube through your anus into your large intestine. This tube allows your doctor to look for signs of disease, take tissue samples for biopsy, and remove any polyps.

48 A *Flexible Sigmoidoscopy* Allows Your Doctor to Examine Your Rectum and the Lower Part of Your Colon

The pretest preparation for a flexible sigmoidoscopy is similar to that for a colonoscopy. However, no sedation is necessary. During the procedure, a short, lighted tube is inserted into the lower part of your colon, which allows your doctor to examine the area, take tissue samples, and remove polyps.

49 An *Upper Endoscopy* Allows Your Doctor to Examine the Upper Parts of Your Digestive Tract

In this test, your doctor uses a flexible lighted tube to take a look at your esophagus, stomach, and duodenum, which is the upper part of your small intestine. You will be asked to fast for a period of time before the procedure, and you will be sedated during the procedure.

50 An *Upper GI Series* Is a Series of X-Rays of Your Upper Digestive System

As in an upper endoscopy, you will be asked to fast before the test. You will then be required to drink a barium solution, which provides contrast for the x-rays. During the procedure, you will be asked to change positions so that multiple pictures can be obtained.

51 A *Barium Enema* Allows for X-Rays to Be Taken of Your Large Intestine

As in a colonoscopy, you will be required to fast and take enemas the day before this procedure. During the procedure a barium solution will be inserted in your rectum to provide contrast for the x-rays. Similar to an upper GI series, you will be asked to shift positions throughout the procedure so that multiple images can be taken.

Medical Treatment Options

52 Don't Agree to Surgery without a Second Opinion

Research has shown that IBS patients are at higher risk for unnecessary surgery, including removal of the gallbladder, appendix, uterus, and all or parts of the large intestine. IBS does not require or necessarily benefit from any type of surgery. Therefore surgery should only be undertaken if diagnostic testing and a second opinion indicate the presence of a more serious medical condition.

53 Learn about the Various Types of Medications Prescribed to Treat the Symptoms of IBS

Unlike many health problems, there is no one medication available to "cure" the problem. Instead, most of the prescription options for IBS are designed to target certain symptoms. There are some new "gut-directed" medications, many of them still in development, that have been formulated specifically for IBS. Knowing what your medication options are can help you to work collaboratively with your doctor to devise an optimal treatment plan.

54 Antispasmodics Are Given to Reduce Pain and Cramping

Because antispasmodics can help ease IBS pain, they tend to be a popular choice for doctors when working with IBS patients. Antispasmodics relax and soothe the smooth muscle lining the intestinal tract, providing relief from abdominal cramping and spasms.

55 You Don't Have to Be Depressed to Benefit from an Antidepressant

Antidepressants can reduce IBS pain and have a beneficial effect on the speed of the muscle contractions of your colon. They are typically prescribed to IBS patients at lower levels than those used for the treatment of depression. Your doctor will choose which type of antidepressant to prescribe depending on whether your primary IBS symptom is constipation or diarrhea.

56 Antibiotics Are Used When SIBO Is Thought to Be Present

As we discussed in Chapter 1, SIBO is thought to be the reason behind IBS in a certain subset of patients. SIBO is treated through the use of certain antibiotics that are not absorbed by your stomach and thus are available to act on any bacteria that might be found in your small intestine.

57 Gut-Directed Medications, Designed Specifically for IBS, Are Starting to Become Available

The medications in this class are designed to directly affect the workings of your large intestine in order to bring about symptom relief. Some of these medications have been withdrawn from the market due to serious side effects. At the time of this writing there are two medications from this class approved for the treatment of IBS-C and one medication approved for the treatment of IBS-D. Other options are still in the development and testing phases.

58 If You Experience Regular Bathroom Accidents (Fecal Incontinence), There Is a Prescription Product That Might Help

Solesta works by building up your anal tissue, helping it to better retain fecal matter. Ask your doctor if you might be a candidate for this treatment.

When to Call Your Doctor

59 Ask Your Doctor about Emergency Coverage

Don't wait until an emergency happens to find out how available your doctor might be when you most need medical care. Find out in advance how to reach your doctor should you have concerns after office hours.

60 Get to Know Which GI Symptoms Should Be Brought to Your Doctor's Attention Immediately

Call your doctor if you experience any of the following symptoms alongside your IBS:

- A sudden change in the nature of your diarrhea symptoms
- A fever that is over 100°F
- Fever that lasts longer than three days
- A sudden change in the nature of your IBS pain
- Any signs of rectal bleeding or blood in the stool
- Vomiting that doesn't stop
- Any other symptom that makes you feel that something is seriously wrong

IBS and the Emergency Room

61 Know When to Go

IBS symptoms can be quite severe and disabling at times. It can be hard to know if what you are experiencing is an IBS attack or some other medical problem. Ask your doctor what signs and symptoms would warrant a call to the office or a trip to the emergency room (ER) or an urgent care center. If in doubt, call or just go.

62 Bring Someone with You

Your experience in the ER will be greatly enhanced if you can bring a friend or family member. They can help reassure you and keep you company while you are waiting. They can also act as your advocate if you feel that your concerns are being dismissed as "only IBS."

63 Know What to Bring Along

To help your visit to go more smoothly, be sure to have the following things with you:

- Health insurance information
- Your doctor's contact information
- A list of your medications and allergies

64 Be Clear and Calm While Describing Your Symptoms

The likelihood that your symptoms will be taken seriously by hospital staff will be greater if you remain calm as you discuss your symptoms and concerns. Now is not the time to be embarrassed—do not be modest in describing your symptoms.

65 Wait Your Turn

You can use the relaxation exercises that you will learn in Chapter 12 to keep yourself calm until the staff is able to offer you some relief. Rather than becoming agitated that you have not yet been seen, see it as a sign that they have assessed your symptoms as being non–life threatening.

66 Be Respectful. . .

Although you may be frightened and in pain, don't forget your manners. Treat staff with appreciation and kindness to maximize the care you receive.

67 ..But Don't Be Afraid to Advocate for Yourself

Don't worry about being a bother. If your symptoms worsen while you are waiting to be attended to, let a staff member know. If you feel that a staff member is not taking your concerns seriously, ask to speak with a supervisor.

Alternative Treatment Options

Because traditional medicine offers limited options for adequate symptom relief, alternatives are frequently sought by people who have IBS. Acquaint yourself with some of the more popular treatments and remedies to see which ones may be helpful for you.

Mind–Body Treatments

68 Mind–Body Treatments Are Often Helpful, and You Don't Have to Worry about Side Effects

Although IBS is not *caused* by stress, it certainly can be worsened when you are under stress. Mind–body treatments are often recommended for IBS patients because they are very good at offsetting the effects of stress. These treatments may also help address any brain–gut dysfunction that is adding to symptoms.

69 If You Are under a Lot of Stress, You May Want to Seek Psychotherapy

There is research that supports the effectiveness of two particular forms of psychotherapy in reducing IBS symptoms. If you choose to try one of these treatments, make sure that the practitioner is licensed or certified.

1. Cognitive behavioral therapy (CBT) involves challenging unhealthy ways of thinking and learning new coping behaviors.
2. Gut-directed hypnotherapy involves being inducted into a trance state during which suggestions are made that address your symptomatology.

70 Acupuncture May (or May Not) Be Helpful for IBS Pain

Acupuncture involves having small needles placed at specific points all over the body. Although some people have reported IBS relief through acupuncture, research on the subject has been mixed.

71 Meditation Can Be Effective for Stress Relief

Some preliminary research supports the effectiveness of meditation in easing IBS symptoms, and a much larger body of research shows that meditation is quite effective in counteracting the effects of psychosocial stress on the body. Unlike medications, meditation offers potential benefits without the risk of serious side effects. Therefore, you may want to consider adding some form of meditation to your regular routine. There are many ways to practice meditation, all with the goal of calming and quieting the mind. You can learn how to practice meditation from a teacher, through reading about different practices, or by listening to audio recordings.

72 Sitting Meditation Helps to Calm an Anxious Mind

Sitting meditation requires that you sit quietly for a period of time. There are many different ways to practice sitting meditation. Trying to pay attention to your breath is one of the simplest. Meditation is not about emptying your mind, but about trying to increase your focus on the present. Like any skill, it takes practice to build up the amount of time that you are able to sit still. You can start by setting a timer for five minutes and counting your inhalations and exhalations. Your mind will run all over the place—that is normal. Just keep bringing your attention back to focus on your breath.

73 Mindfulness Helps to Keep You More Focused on the Present

Our busy minds like to constantly review the past and worry about the future. Mindfulness practice is a way to improve your ability to be present in the here and now. A sitting meditative practice will help with this, but you can also practice paying attention to what you are actually doing as you go through your day. Sometimes it helps to start small; for example, to truly focus on the foods you are eating or to try to pay full attention as you brush your teeth in the morning. You will learn some strategies for improved mindfulness in Chapter 12.

74 Yoga Is a Movement-Based Form of Meditation

As with meditation, some preliminary research indicates that practicing yoga can help ease the symptoms of IBS. Through its emphasis on breath work, as well as practices that stretch and strengthen the body, yoga can be very calming. It provides a wonderful counterbalance to the stress of modern life and the stress of having a chronic health problem like IBS. Although a wide variety of yoga instructional videos is available, there are benefits in learning directly from a qualified yoga instructor so as to reduce the risk of injury.

75 Tai Chi Is an Alternative Form of Moving Meditation

Unlike meditation and yoga, there is to date no solid research regarding the benefits of tai chi for IBS. However, like yoga, tai chi is a moving form of meditation that has excellent stress-relieving qualities. Tai chi involves a series of gentle movements that provide a nice low-impact option for physical calming.

Alternative Physical Treatments

76 Biofeedback May Be Helpful for Constipation

Biofeedback is a treatment in which sensors are used to help train you to use the muscles of your pelvic floor and anus more efficiently. This is a good treatment option for anyone who has severe constipation caused by a condition known as dyssynergic defecation. In this condition, the muscles responsible for enabling a bowel movement do not work as they should.

77 Physical Therapy Is Another Option for Problems with Chronic Constipation

In the past, Kegel exercises were routinely recommended to patients who have dyssynergic defecation or have experienced fecal incontinence (soiling). However, this is no longer the case. The current thinking is that it is more helpful to relax and stretch the muscles of the pelvic floor. If you think this sounds like a good option for you, look for a physical therapist who specializes in this area.

Over-the-Counter Remedies (OTCs)

78 OTCs Can Offer Immediate Symptom Relief or Work over a Longer Period to Ease Symptoms

There is such a wide variety of OTCs available for addressing IBS symptoms! Taking a few moments to learn about some of the more common options can help you assess whether or not a particular OTC would be of help to you. Remember, just because something is sold without a prescription does not necessarily make it a safe option. Before trying any new OTC, be sure to check with your doctor first.

79 Peppermint Oil Can Be Effective in Easing the Painful Spasms of IBS

Peppermint oil has strong research support in terms of its effectiveness for IBS. In fact, peppermint oil may be just as effective as prescription antispasmodics. If you decide to try peppermint oil (and your doctor says it's okay), choose an enteric-coated capsule to minimize the risk of experiencing heartburn as a side effect.

80 Slippery Elm Is an Age-Old Remedy for Digestive Woes

Slippery elm is an herbal remedy, available in capsule or powder form. It is thought to calm gut inflammation, and to both soften and add bulk to the stool, thus making it helpful for easing both constipation and diarrhea. There is no direct research support for the use of slippery elm for IBS, but it is generally considered to be a safe option.

81 Digestive Enzyme Supplements Are Thought to Enhance Digestion

As a normal part of digestion the pancreas releases enzymes that help break down the components of the foods we eat. Digestive enzyme supplements are thought to augment the action of these naturally occurring enzymes. Again, there is no research to show that such supplements help in IBS, but they do not seem to be harmful.

OTCs for Constipation

82 For Constipation, Think about Triphala

Triphala is an herbal preparation used in Ayurvedic medicine, a centuries-old Hindu system of medicine. The preparation consists of powdered forms of three dried fruits from the amalaki, bibhataki, and haritaki trees. Triphala has a laxative effect and is thought to also reduce abdominal pain and bloating. It is also a great source of antioxidants, substances that have been shown to reduce your risk of cancer.

83 A Magnesium Supplement May Also Help Ease Constipation

Magnesium has long been known to have a laxative effect. In fact, magnesium is a primary ingredient in most colonoscopy prep formulations. When taking it as a supplement, be sure to follow the manufacturer's instructions for dosing. Also be aware that magnesium supplements may interfere with the effectiveness of other medications that you may be taking. If you choose to try a magnesium supplement be sure to inform your doctor.

84 Learn about Fiber Supplements

Fiber supplements, sometimes called bulk laxatives, are products that you take to increase your intake of dietary fiber. This is typically recommended as a way to ease constipation. If you choose to try a fiber supplement, start out slowly to allow your body time to adjust and to reduce the risk of gas and bloating.

85 Psyllium (Ispaghula Husk) for IBS-C

Psyllium is a plant-based source of soluble fiber sold under a variety of names. The American College of Gastroenterology has concluded that soluble fiber may be better for constipation management than insoluble fiber, making psyllium a helpful option for anyone with IBS-C.

86 Calcium Polycarbophil Carries Less Risk of Causing Intestinal Gas

Calcium polycarbophil is a synthetic form of fiber that has been found to be less likely than other fiber supplement products to cause unwanted gas and bloating. Calcium polycarbophil is also sold under several brand names.

87 Methylcellulose Is a Good Choice for Anyone Following the Low-FODMAP Diet

Found in the product Citrucel, methylcellulose is composed of both synthetic and natural fiber. Citrucel is recommended for those on a low-FODMAP diet (see Chapter 7) because it does not result in fermentation by gut bacteria.

88 Learn about Osmotic Laxatives

Osmotic laxatives work by increasing the amount of water in the large intestine, helping to keep stools moist and making them easier to pass. The osmotic laxatives Miralax and Lactulose are considered by the American College of Gastroenterology to be safe and effective for the treatment of constipation. Milk of magnesia is also an osmotic laxative, but it carries some health risks and does not have research support for its effectiveness.

89 Stool Softeners Can Offer Temporary Relief of Constipation

Stool softeners do just what their name implies—they work to soften stool so as to help initiate a bowel movement. They are generally only recommended for short-term use. Be sure to drink plenty of water when taking stool softeners.

90 Use Caution When Using Herbal Stimulant Laxatives

Herbal stimulant laxatives consist of preparations containing herbs like senna and cascara sagrada. There have been some safety concerns with laxatives in this class and they tend to carry the risk of unwanted side effects. If you do choose to use an herbal stimulant laxative, do not take it for more than one week.

OTCs for Diarrhea

91 A Calcium Supplement May Help Reduce Diarrhea Episodes

Many IBS patients swear that taking a calcium supplement has been helpful for their IBS-D. Calcium supplements can interfere with other medications, so be sure to discuss the idea with your doctor. Absorption of calcium is best when the dosage is below 500 milligrams, so you may need to take the supplement several times throughout the day.

92 It's Okay to Reach for the Imodium

Imodium is generally considered to be a safe and effective OTC option for calming diarrhea. Be sure to follow the manufacturer's or your doctor's recommendation regarding dosage amounts. The one drawback of Imodium that many people with IBS report is that it can work too well, resulting in constipation. (If you have inflammatory bowel disease [IBD], check with your doctor before taking Imodium.)

OTCs for Gas and Bloating

93 Probiotic Supplements Seem to Offer a Safe Option for Reducing Gas and Other IBS Symptoms

Probiotic supplements contain strains of so-called friendly bacteria—bacteria that have been shown to have a favorable effect on our health. Probiotics are generally considered to be safe, with a very low risk of negative side effects. Look for a brand that contains a high number of live organisms. If you don't notice a favorable effect on your IBS symptoms within one month, you may want to try a different brand.

94 Try a Gas-Reducing Product

Beano is a supplement that contains digestive enzymes. These enzymes break down complex sugars in foods so that they cannot be fermented by bacteria in the large intestine. Gas-X (simethicone) works by breaking up gas bubbles in the digestive tract.

95 If You Are Lactose Intolerant, Consider a Lactase Supplement

These supplements add the digestive enzyme lactase to the digestive tract, thus enabling people who have lactose intolerance to fully digest the sugar lactose found in dairy products. This means that a person who is lactose intolerant may be able to eat some dairy products without unwanted symptoms such as gas, bloating, and diarrhea.

Eating with IBS

For years, doctors and researchers minimized the effects of food on IBS symptoms. This was in sharp contrast to the experience of people who actually had the disorder! Luckily, the times have changed and there is much more information available as to the role that food plays in IBS. Changing what you eat may not only help you avoid exacerbating symptoms but also may be a way to prevent symptoms in the first place.

General Eating Tips

96 Eat Whole Foods

Whole foods are foods that are minimally processed—foods that contain ingredients that you can readily recognize. Avoid eating processed convenience foods that contain things like preservatives, artificial coloring, and artificial flavorings. If you don't know what something is, neither will your digestive system.

97 Cook at Home

You will be doing your digestive and overall health a great service if you learn to enjoy home cooking. When you do the cooking you have more control over the quality of the foods that you are eating, as well as the ingredients in each dish.

98 Avoid Foods with Unhealthy Fats

Foods that are greasy or fried can strengthen intestinal contractions, causing painful cramps and urgent diarrhea. This means no more fried chicken, French fries, and heavy gravies. You may miss some of these favorite foods, but your colon won't!

99 Eat Foods That Have Healthy Fats

Many people eat a diet that is deficient in super-healthy omega-3 fatty acids. These healthy fats are anti-inflammatory and appear to be good for the health of your brain as well as your gut. Try to incorporate the following foods into your daily diet:

- Avocados
- Coconut oil
- Nuts and nut butters
- Olives and olive oil
- Fish, such as anchovies, salmon, and sardines

100 You May Find That You Tolerate Vegetables and Fruits Better When They Are Cooked

Many people who have IBS find that they have a hard time tolerating raw vegetables and fruits, yet can handle the same foods when they are cooked. It may be that the cooking process helps to break down fiber, making it easier for your digestive system to handle.

101 Don't Eat Too Much at One Sitting

Meals that are too large can also intensify the strength of intestinal contractions. Keep your portion sizes reasonable. You may find that it is better to eat small meals throughout the day, rather than sticking to three large meals. The only exception to this rule is if you are being treated for SIBO. If that it is the case, it is better to stick to three meals with several hours in between. This will take better advantage of the small intestine's natural cleansing wave, which operates between meals.

102 Don't Skip Meals

Many people who have IBS skip meals to try to prevent experiencing symptoms while they are out of the house. The problem with this strategy is that eating intermittently can contribute to motility dysfunction. You want to think of your digestive tract as a conveyor belt. In order for it to operate smoothly, it needs to receive food at regular, predictable times. In addition, skipping meals can leave you at risk for overeating when you finally give yourself permission to eat. Overeating can then trigger the very symptoms you were trying to prevent.

103 Start to Eat More Fermented Foods

When certain foods are subjected to a fermenting process, the resulting product is filled with helpful bacteria and enzymes. Eating fermented foods is an excellent way to bring natural sources of probiotics into your system, with a wider variety of strains than can be found in a probiotic supplement. Here are some examples:

- Fermented vegetables, including fresh sauerkraut and kimchi
- Fermented drinks, including kefir and kombucha
- Yogurt

104 Eat More Prebiotics

Prebiotics are components of ordinary foods that stimulate the growth of beneficial gut bacteria. Some IBS-friendly sources of prebiotics include bananas and blueberries. Unfortunately, many of the foods that serve as good sources of prebiotics are also high in FODMAPs, which you will learn more about in Chapter 7. You can experiment with eating the following foods in small portions to see if you can tolerate them without making your symptoms worse:

- Asparagus
- Garlic
- Jerusalem artichokes
- Leeks
- Onions
- Wheat
- Rye

105 Whenever Possible, Choose Organic or Locally Grown Produce

Conventionally grown vegetables and fruits are often grown in depleted soil and drenched in pesticides. Although there is no research to tie such produce to IBS, you know that you have a sensitive digestive system, so why risk it? Organic produce may cost more, but your health is worth it. Locally grown produce is another option, as small farmers tend to use less pesticide than large growers. Smaller farms generally use traditional farming techniques such as crop rotation and composting to keep their plants healthy.

106 Cut Back on Sugar and Foods with Refined Carbohydrates

Modern diets have become overloaded with sugar and refined carbohydrates, most notably white flour. Although foods containing these ingredients are convenient, they are rarely healthy and nutritious. The carbohydrate load from sugar and from flour that has had its fiber removed can contribute to an unhealthy balance of gut flora and thus unwanted digestive symptoms.

Best Teas

107 Reach for a Soothing Cup of Tea

When your IBS is acting up, sipping on a hot cup of tea can be quite soothing. Be sure to choose a tea that is right for your symptoms.

108 Peppermint Tea Is Thought to Have Anti-Spasmodic Benefits

Peppermint tea is your best option regardless of what your predominant IBS symptoms are. Peppermint tea is thought to soothe IBS pain, calm intestinal cramping, and relieve gas and bloating.

109 Anise Tea Is a Good Option if You Are Constipated

Anise tea is thought to have laxative properties as well as to provide relief of gas and bloating. It has a pleasant licorice-like flavor.

110 Fennel Tea Is Another Good Option for Constipation

Fennel tea is also thought to be helpful for easing constipation, as well as relieving abdominal pain and intestinal spasms. However, fennel tea is not appropriate for anyone on the low-FODMAP diet.

111 Chamomile Tea Is a Soothing Option for Calming Diarrhea

Chamomile tea is thought to provide a calming effect on the central nervous system and to help quiet intestinal cramping. Unfortunately, chamomile tea is not appropriate for the low-FODMAP diet.

Green Juices and Smoothies

112 Vegetable Juices and Green Smoothies Offer a Way to Increase Your Intake of Fruits and Vegetables

In our modern world, it can be hard to take in enough plant-based foods to meet our dietary needs. One option you can explore is to see how your body reacts if you drink your produce through the use of a juicer or blender.

113 Juicing Your Fruits and Vegetables Allows for a Quick Influx of Nutrients

A juicer pulls out the liquid from fruits and vegetables, leaving behind the pulp. Without the fibrous pulp, the micronutrients in the produce can be quickly absorbed by the body into the bloodstream. Again, there is no research on the benefits of juicing for IBS. but since juicing appears to take out the harder-to-digest insoluble fiber while still allowing intake of the better-for-IBS soluble fiber, juicing may be something for you to explore.

114 Green Smoothies Allow You to Benefit Fully from the Fiber in Produce

Smoothies are created by putting fresh fruits and vegetables through a blender. This means that you are getting all of the gut-healthy fiber that they contain. IBS-friendly supplements such as chia seeds and flaxseed can easily be added to smoothies.

115 To Maximize Success When New to Juicing or Green Smoothies, Start with Low-FODMAP Produce Options

Choosing low-FODMAP fruits and vegetables when first adding vegetable juices or green smoothies to your diet may help your gut to adjust to the increase in fiber without exacerbating your symptoms. After a period of time, with your gut flora theoretically being nurtured by all the healthy plant-based foods you are drinking, you may find that you can broaden the range of produce that you can tolerate.

Need to Lose Weight?

116 Cut Out Sugar and White Flour

Sugar and foods made with white flour trigger an insulin response within your body that triggers cravings for more food a short time after eating, sabotaging any efforts to "be good" with your eating. Eating excessive sugar and refined carbohydrates and the resulting insulin response raises your risk for cardiovascular disease, diabetes, and obesity. It may take a few days to kick the habit, but saying no to sugar and refined carbohydrates will become much easier once you eliminate them fully from your diet. You will lose weight and your gut flora will thank you.

117 Load Up on Vegetables

Vegetables are low in calories and high in nourishment. You may choose to start with low-FODMAP veggies until your body adjusts to the higher amounts of dietary fiber that you will be eating. Try to add some vegetables to every meal— have spinach in a breakfast omelet, enjoy vegetable soup or a salad for lunch, and then be sure to fill half your plate with vegetables at dinner.

118 Enjoy Reasonable Amounts of Animal Protein

Alongside your vegetables, feel free to fill your belly with protein. Protein is generally well digested and does not trigger the insulin response that leads to food cravings. When possible, choose humanely raised, pastured or grass-fed products to reduce your exposure to unhealthy toxins. Good sources of animal protein include:

- Chicken
- Fish
- Pork
- Turkey
- Lean cuts of beef

119 Don't Skimp on Healthy Fats

Although you may have been told that "fats make you fat," there is now increasing evidence that this was a dietary mistake. Eating foods with healthy fats (see Tip 99) will not cause you to gain weight, but rather will make you feel more satisfied in between meals and thus less likely to cheat on your diet. Just be sure to watch your portion size so that you don't go overboard on calories.

120 Go Light on Fruit

While fruit is a wonderful source of nutrition, too much of it can derail your weight loss goals. Choose fruit when you are craving a sweet snack, but otherwise don't overdo it.

121 Drink Plenty of Water

Not only is water good for avoiding constipation or becoming dehydrated by diarrhea episodes, it also is a great weight-loss tool. Often, we reach for food when really all our bodies are asking for is hydration. Before choosing to eat an unplanned snack, drink a full glass of water first to see if that sates you enough to make it to your next meal.

122 Move Your Body

Try to find some form of exercise that your body enjoys and can tolerate. This does not have to be formal exercise—dancing around your house and taking the stairs instead of the elevator all count. You may want to incorporate some strength training into your weekly routine to tone up muscle and increase your metabolism. Don't despair if IBS prevents you from regularly exercising. Weight loss is more likely to come from dietary change than from exercise. You will find more tips for incorporating physical exercise into your life in Chapter 13.

Need to Gain Weight?

123 Consider Eating Four Meals a Day

Rather than stick to the conventional breakfast, lunch, and dinner schedule, plan to have four meals each day. Eating more frequently not only may help you to take in more calories, but also may help your digestive tract to move its contents along more smoothly.

124 Eat One More Snack after Dinner

You may be able to sneak in a few extras calories if you plan for a somewhat substantial snack a few hours after you have eaten dinner. Just don't eat too close to bedtime, particularly if you are at risk for acid reflux.

125 Incorporate More Healthy Fats into Your Diet

If you are trying to gain weight, feel free to eat as much as you want of those foods with healthy fats that are listed in Tip 99. Reach for nuts and nut butters for snacks, add avocados to your salads, and try coconut oil in your smoothies.

Eating for Symptom Relief

There is no one-size-fits-all approach that works for IBS. You may need to employ different dietary strategies depending on which IBS symptoms you are currently experiencing. In this chapter, we will cover eating tips tailored to some of the more common IBS symptoms.

Eating Tips for Constipation

126 Eat a Big Breakfast

For most people, natural biorhythms are such that the body would prefer to eliminate in the morning. You can work with your body's inner clock by making sure to eat a large breakfast, preferably with some healthy fat content, in order to initiate a bowel movement.

127 Drinking a Cup of Coffee Can Help Get Things Going

If you found that coffee helps to stimulate a bowel movement, you are not imagining things. Scientists are not completely sure why this happens, but it does appear that there is some substance within coffee that triggers the urge for evacuation. One thing they know is that caffeine is not the reason as decaffeinated coffee has the same effect.

128 Add Flaxseed to Your Daily Diet

Flaxseed can help keep your stools soft and moist, thus making them easier to pass. Flaxseed is considered to be an excellent source of dietary fiber and omega-3 fatty acids. Flaxseeds need to be ground before eating, which can be done with the help of a small coffee grinder. Once they are ground, flaxseed must be refrigerated. Flaxseed has a pleasant, nutty taste—add it to smoothies or sprinkle on yogurt. Be sure to drink plenty of water when eating flaxseed.

129 Chia Seeds Are Another Good Option for Softening Stools

These little poppy-seed–size seeds are also a good source of fiber and omega-3 fatty acids. Unlike flaxseed, chia seeds can be eaten whole. Chia seeds can be added to smoothies, made into a pudding, or soaked and added to oatmeal.

130 Make Sure You Are Taking in Enough Dietary Fiber

Fiber is the part of plant food that cannot be digested. Fiber provides bulk and moisture to the stool and facilitates a healthy balance of gut microflora, thus encouraging regular bowel movements. For most adults, adequate fiber intake is approximately 20 to 25 milligrams a day. To make sure you get adequate amounts of fiber be sure to eat plenty of vegetables, fruits, and, if tolerated, whole grains and legumes. It is best to slowly increase the amount of fiber you consume to minimize any reactive gastrointestinal symptoms.

131 Drink Plenty of Water

Every cell in our bodies needs water in order to function optimally. When we don't drink enough water, our body pulls water from fecal matter in the intestines. This results in hard stools that are more difficult to pass.

Eating Tips for Diarrhea

132 Eat Light Meals Throughout Your Day

A large, heavy meal can intensify the strength of intestinal cramping, leading to pain and continued emptying. Keep your meals light and small, and try to avoid anything creamy, fried, or greasy.

133 Don't Skip Meals

Many people who suffer from IBS-D tend to make the mistake of thinking that if they skip meals they can avoid episodes. However, you already know that your digestive system works in fits and starts. You can help ease your body onto a more normal rhythm by eating your meals on a regular, consistent schedule.

134 Avoid Artificial Sweeteners

Many sugar substitutes, particularly those ending in "-ol," have a laxative effect on the body, which is the last thing you need if your body is prone to diarrhea episodes. Because of how they interact with gut bacteria, they can also contribute to gas and bloating. Therefore, it is best to avoid sugar-free foods, drinks, and chewing gums.

135 Avoid Dairy Food

Even if you have not been diagnosed with lactose intolerance, you may want to think about cutting out dairy food altogether. Research suggests that a high number of people who have IBS are unable to digest lactose. You can meet your calcium needs by making sure that you eat plenty of vegetables, especially green leafy types.

Eating Tips for Alternating Type IBS (IBS-A)

136 Make Sure to Eat Your Meals on a Regular Schedule

If you find that you alternate between constipation and diarrhea, the conveyor belt that is your digestive tract is not moving smoothly. Just as in IBS-D, eating your meals at regular, predictable intervals can help your body to find a more regular rhythm.

137 Slowly Add More Fiber to Your Diet, Paying Attention to Both Soluble and Insoluble Fiber Intake

Soluble fiber dissolves in water, keeping stool matter soft. Insoluble fiber does not absorb water and therefore helps to keep stool and your intestines lubricated. Bulking up the stool with fiber may help ensure a more predictable pattern of bowel movements. Eating a wide variety of vegetables and fruits (low-FODMAP if necessary), will ensure a healthy intake of both types of fiber.

Eating Tips for Gas and Bloating

138 Don't Chew Gum

Believe it or not, the simple act of chewing gum can increase intestinal gas and bloating. When we chew gum, we are likely to swallow air. That air has to come out somehow!

139 Eat Your Meals Slowly

You know that old expression, "Don't gulp your meal"? It is still good advice. Taking the time to eat slowly helps to ensure that you are not taking in excessive amounts of air along with your food.

140 Avoid Carbonated Beverages

The process of carbonation results in air bubbles within beverages—air that can make its way down into the intestines. So avoid soda and beer. Drink water instead!

141 Limit FODMAPs

As we have discussed, FODMAPs are carbohydrates found in ordinary foods. One of the reasons that FODMAPs cause problems for people with IBS is that they can be highly fermentable. The fermentation process can result in problematic intestinal gas for people who have IBS. Whether or not you choose to be on a low-FODMAP diet, you may find that you experience less intestinal gas when you minimize your intake of foods that are high in FODMAPs on the days when you really, really need to be gas free.

Special IBS Diets

There is increasing evidence that a comprehensive dietary approach may help alleviate IBS symptoms. However, just as IBS can present itself differently in different people, a dietary approach that works for one person may not work for the next. Here you will learn about some of the more common IBS dietary approaches: the gluten-free diet, the low-FODMAP diet, the elimination diet, and a grain-free diet. Remember to always check with your doctor before making any kind of substantial dietary change.

Tips for Success on a Special Diet

142 Tell Others

It will be much easier to be successful in following a special diet if you tell the people you are with what your dietary needs are. You don't need to go into great detail; just let them know what food options are open and closed to you because of your condition.

143 Read Labels Carefully

Do your best to eat whole foods whenever possible. If you choose to eat a prepared food, check the label to ensure that there are no hidden ingredients that might set your system off.

144 Separate Out Foods That You Can and Cannot Eat

Keep temptation out of harm's way. You have three options: throw away, give away, or store separately any foods that are not appropriate for your diet.

145 Keep Appropriate Snacks Available

Make a list of take-along snack foods and be sure you have some available to you at all times. These snacks will serve you well when out and about in case your choices for finding appropriate foods are limited. Such snacks will be essential when traveling, as often your only options will be gut-unhealthy fast food. These snacks can also serve to fill your belly if you are at a social event with limited food options that you can enjoy and tolerate.

146 Work with a Qualified Dietary Professional

It can be challenging to try to eat differently from the majority of the population. Working with a health coach or dietitian can help you remain on track. These professionals can also help you find recipes and plan your meals, as well as develop strategies for navigating through challenging situations.

The Gluten-Free Diet

147 You Can Have a Sensitivity to Gluten Even If You Don't Have Celiac Disease

It is possible to experience gastrointestinal or other non-GI symptoms in response to gluten even if you do not have celiac disease. Although the mechanisms behind gluten sensitivity are not clearly understood, many people with IBS have found relief from their symptoms once they have removed gluten from their diets.

148 Don't Go Gluten Free without Being Tested for Celiac Disease First

As discussed in Chapter 1, people who have IBS are at a higher risk for celiac disease and therefore should be tested for the disease. Since the testing is only accurate if you are eating gluten, do not attempt a gluten-free diet until you have completed celiac disease testing. (Remember, people with celiac disease can never eat anything containing gluten as they put themselves at risk for serious health complications.)

149 A Gluten Sensitivity Is Identified through the Use of an Elimination Diet

If you think that gluten may be contributing to your symptoms, you can find out for sure by avoiding anything that contains gluten for at least four weeks. If you see an improvement at the end of that period, gluten may be a problem for you.

150 Gluten Is a Protein Found in Wheat, Rye, and Barley

To go gluten free, you will have to give up eating and drinking anything that contains gluten. This includes cereals, bread, and baked goods made with gluten-containing ingredients, and drinks such as some brands of beer, soda, and hot chocolate. You will also have to read labels carefully, as gluten is frequently used as a food additive.

151 Gluten-Free Processed Foods Are Convenient but May Not Be the Healthiest of Choices

To make their products more appealing, many processed food manufacturers add excessive amounts of sugars, fats, and other ingredients. These products also tend to lack nutrients and vitamins.

152 Eating Whole Foods Is a Healthy Way to Go Gluten Free

Unprocessed vegetables, fruits, meat, poultry, and fish are all foods that are naturally gluten free. These foods are filled with healthy nutrients and you can eat them freely without having to worry that they contain hidden ingredients and gluten.

153 Have Fun Exploring Alternative, Gluten-Free Grains

With experimentation you may find that you can enjoy gluten-free versions of your favorite foods. The following grains are all gluten free:

- Amaranth
- Buckwheat
- Corn
- Millet
- Oats (look for those marked gluten-free)
- Quinoa
- Rice and wild rice
- Sorghum
- Teff

154 A Gluten Challenge Is Just as Important as the Gluten Elimination

Before you can conclude that gluten is problematic for you, you need to re-expose yourself to gluten and assess your symptoms. This step is important to make sure that it is really the gluten-free diet that has helped and not some other factor. This re-exposure is called a *challenge*.

155 For the Gluten Challenge, Pick a Time When it Would Not Be Too Inconvenient for You to Experience Symptoms

On the day of your challenge, eat a small portion of a food that contains gluten. On the next day, eat a few items that contain gluten. If you experience a resumption of your previous digestive symptoms after eating gluten, you can conclude that you appear to have gluten sensitivity.

The Low-FODMAP Diet

156 **The Low-FODMAP Diet Is the Only Dietary Approach with Research Support for its Effectiveness in Treating IBS**

The low-FODMAP diet was developed by researchers from Monash University in Australia. Several studies suggest that it offers significant symptom relief to approximately three-quarters of IBS patients who follow the diet.

157 **FODMAPs Are Types of Carbohydrates Found in Ordinary Foods**

FODMAPs stands for Fermentable Oligosaccharides, Disaccharides, Monosaccharides, and Polyols. They can be found in a variety of foods, including fruits, vegetables, and whole grains.

158 **Ideally, the Diet Should Be Undertaken under the Supervision of a Qualified Dietary Professional**

The diet can be tricky because high-FODMAP ingredients such as onions, garlic, and wheat are found in many of the foods that people typically eat. A qualified professional can ensure that you are taking in adequate nutrition while on the diet and help you to identify which FODMAPs are troublesome for you.

159 **The Initial Phase of the Diet Requires That You Only Eat Foods That Are Low in FODMAPs**

In the initial phase of the diet, called the Elimination phase, you would avoid high-FODMAP foods and only consume low-FODMAP foods. This phase should last approximately four to eight weeks.

160 The Monash University Low-FODMAP Diet App Is a Great Resource

Although FODMAP food lists can be found online, many of them contain conflicting information. This is because not every food has been tested for its FODMAP content. Monash University has developed an app for mobile devices that offers up-to-date lab-tested information on the FODMAP content of common foods.

161 There Are Five Types of FODMAPs

Researchers have broken down the classification of FODMAPs into five types. Not every person is reactive to every FODMAP type:

1. *Fructans* are classified as oligosaccharides and can be found in wheat, many vegetables (most notably garlic and onions), and the food additives fructooligosaccharide (FOS) and inulin.
2. *GOS* stands for galactooligosaccharides, which are sometimes called galactans. GOS are found primarily in legumes, including beans, chickpeas, and lentils.
3. *Lactose* is a disaccharide. You are probably already acquainted with lactose and may even have self-identified a lactose intolerance. Lactose, as you most likely know, is found in many dairy products. However, the lactose level in some dairy items, such as some cheeses, is low enough that these items can be appropriate for a low-FODMAP diet.
4. *Fructose* is a monosaccharide. Fructose is the sugar found in many fruits, honey, and the seemingly ever-present high fructose corn syrup (HCFS).
5. *Polyols* are sugar alcohols with scientific names that typically end in "-ol." Polyols are found naturally in some fruits, such as blackberries, and vegetables such as cauliflower

and mushrooms. In addition, many artificial sweeteners contain polyols.

162 The Initial Phase of the Low-FODMAP Diet Requires You to Eat Gluten Free, but Not Because of the Gluten

Foods made with wheat, rye, and barley are not allowed during the elimination phase of the diet, not because of their gluten content, but because of their *fructan* content. In fact, some researchers believe that what IBS patients describe as gluten sensitivity may really be a FODMAP sensitivity.

163 After the Initial Elimination Phase, It Is Essential That You Test Each FODMAP Type to Assess Your Own Individual Triggers

In the second phase of the diet, known as the challenge phase, you will systematically try out each type of FODMAP and assess the effect of that FODMAP on your symptoms. Identifying the specific FODMAP types that you are reactive to can help you to eat as wide a variety of food as you can tolerate. A qualified dietary professional can offer you support and guidance as you navigate through this phase.

164 The Low-FODMAP Diet May Result in "Gut Healing"

It is possible that after finishing the elimination phase of the diet that you may be able to tolerate foods that you weren't able to tolerate before starting the diet. In addition, you should periodically rechallenge the FODMAPs you have identified as troublesome to see if your tolerance has improved.

165 The More FODMAPs You Eat in a Sitting or a Day, the More Likely You Are to Have Digestive Symptoms

Keeping in mind this notion of "FODMAP load," you may find that you can tolerate some high-FODMAP foods in small amounts. Eat too many, too soon, and you may become symptomatic.

166 FODMAPs Are Not Unhealthy Foods

Many high FODMAP foods are healthy, nutritious foods. Some of them are classified as prebiotics, which are foods that are important for a healthy gut flora.

167 The Low-FODMAP Diet Is Not Intended for Long-Term Use

It is thought that there may be health risks associated with a long-term strict restriction of high-FODMAP foods due to the loss of prebiotic benefits. This makes the challenge phase essential to ensure that you are eating as wide a variety of FODMAP-containing foods as you can tolerate. You should also engage in periodic rechallenging so that you can expand the types of foods you eat over time.

The Elimination Diet

168 An Elimination Diet Can Be Used to Identify Food Sensitivities

Diagnostic testing for food sensitivities is limited. Therefore, such sensitivities are best identified through the use of an elimination diet. Like the gluten-free and low-FODMAP diets, an elimination diet requires you to avoid certain foods for a period of two to eight weeks. The length of the diet depends on your symptoms and your ability to be compliant with the restrictions.

169 Certain Foods Are More Likely to Cause a Food Sensitivity

In an elimination diet, you restrict foods that are most likely to cause a sensitivity. These include:

- Corn
- Dairy
- Eggs
- Gluten
- Peanuts
- Shellfish
- Soy

170 At the End of the Elimination Phase, You Slowly Reintroduce Each Food in a Systematic Way in Order to Figure Out Which Foods Your Body Is Reactive To

Once the elimination phase is over, you will test each food group one at a time. Pick one food to start and eat several small portions of that food on one day. Don't eat the food on the following two days, but watch to see if your symptoms return. If they do, you can conclude that you have a sensitivity to that food. If you have no symptoms after reintroducing a food to your diet, you can assume that that food is not a trigger for you. After each three-day test, you can start over with the next food group.

Going Grain Free

171 Many People Report That Their IBS Symptoms Cleared Up after Removing All Grains from Their Diet

Although anecdotally people with IBS have reported that their digestive symptoms improved significantly by following a grain-free diet, there is very little research on the subject. Grain-free diet theorists cite research indicating that some substances within grains are harmful for the health of the gut flora, contribute to inflammation, and increase gut fermentation, all of which could theoretically create IBS symptoms.

172 Some Advocates of a Grain-Free Diet Follow a Paleolithic Style of Eating

Paleo diet enthusiasts base their diets on the belief that our ancestors evolved eating only protein and plant foods, with grains entering the picture relatively late in our development. Paleo diet theorists point to the many health problems that have entered into the human condition with the introduction of grains. It should be noted that other scientists have challenged the foundational underpinnings of the Paleo theory.

173 Grain Free May Have Its Downsides

One of the biggest downsides to going grain free is that it can be challenging to try to follow such a diet in a grain-filled world. In addition, some nutrition experts express concerns that a diet excluding grains would not provide enough dietary fiber, vitamins, and minerals. On the other side of the debate, grain-free proponents point out that there is evidence that our early non–grain-eating ancestors were quite healthy. If the idea of this diet appeals to you, discuss the topic with your doctor.

Handling Symptoms

IBS symptoms can have quite a detrimental effect on your quality of life. In this chapter, we will discuss some tried-and-true self-care tips for reducing the pain, motility problems, and discomforts of gas and bloating that are associated with IBS. Incorporating the strategies that seem right for you can help decrease the impact that your digestive system has on your ability to enjoy your life.

Pain Management

174 Use a Heating Pad or Hot Water Bottle

This low-tech, old-fashioned strategy can actually be quite effective. In addition to offering some nice psychological soothing, heat can help relax abdominal muscles, quieting down cramping, and therefore easing pain.

175 Use Guided Imagery

Guided imagery is a mind–body technique that uses the power of your imagination to bring about pain relief. To start, you would close your eyes, focus on your breathing and imagine yourself in a peaceful, beautiful place. Next, you would allow an image to form that represents your pain. For example, you might imagine a flaming ball of fire or a devil poking you with a hot poker. Don't try to force it, just allow whatever image comes to you to pop up. Last, you would start to modify the image in a way that you believe would help ease the pain. Using the above examples, you would imagine spraying the hot ball of fire with a soft spray until the fire starts to subside or imagine that the devil's poker starts to soften into a feather that tickles you. You get the idea.

176 Your Ability to Get Pain Relief from Guided Imagery Will Increase with Practice

Although guided imagery might not be as powerful as, say, morphine, it can help relax muscles and stimulate the brain to send out those pain-reducing chemicals called endorphins. Like any other skill, your attempts at using imagery for pain relief will get better with practice. If nothing else, it gives you something to do and to focus on when your pain gets really bad.

Handling Diarrhea Episodes

177 Use Relaxation Exercises

The calmer you can keep yourself, even at the height of the storm, the more you will be able to help your bowels to quiet down. Keeping in mind the body's own stress response, it is essential that you try to keep your anxiety level low so as not to agitate your digestive tract any more than it already is. Instructions for relaxation exercises can be found in Chapter 12.

178 Use Calming Self-Talk

Due to the mind–body connection, your thoughts can very much affect how you feel. When you think, "Uh-oh, here comes an attack," you could very well be triggering the symptoms you most fear. Here are some things you can say to yourself:

- "It might just be a twinge, let me wait and see what happens."
- "No need to panic. I will just breathe deeply and make my way to the bathroom."
- "Okay, I'm having an episode. Let me just focus on what my body needs to do until it is over."
- "Odds are I will not have an accident. Even though the urges are strong, my sphincter will hold it in until I get to the toilet."
- "No one will judge me because I needed to rush to the bathroom or have been in there for so long. They will just think that I am sick and will have empathy."

179 Don't Try to Empty

It has been my experience that many people are under the mistaken impression that if they fully empty their bowels before leaving the house, they will be less likely to have a problem during the rest of the day. However, there is really no such thing as an empty bowel because fecal matter will continue to replace whatever has been excreted. The problem is that (as you have probably noticed), with each trip to the bathroom, your stools get looser and looser. This is because the fecal matter has not been in the bowels long enough for water to be pulled out. And, unfortunately, our anus is not as good at holding in loose stool, setting you up for the possibility of a bathroom accident.

180 After the Initial One or Two Trips to the Bathroom, Try to Calm Your Body Down

Once you have passed the initial stool that was residing in your rectum, it is not really necessary to continue to empty. Your body may have other ideas about this, but you can try to use relaxation exercises to see if you can quiet down your intestinal spasms without another trip back to the toilet. If the urges become really strong, by all means, go to the bathroom! The point of this tip is that you don't want to actively encourage the emptying, but rather the calming. It would be better if your body retained the loose stool so as to shape it up for a (hopefully!) more normal bowel movement tomorrow.

181 Use Delay When Possible

In addition to using your skills at calming your body when in the middle of a diarrhea episode, you can also use them at other times to see if you can delay those repeated trips to the bathroom. Of course, this will probably not work if your urges are quite strong. However, every mild urge may not signify a real need to empty your rectum. If you have already passed solid or semisolid stool within the past few hours, you may be able to use delay to "hold in" the stool, helping it to firm up for a more productive bowel movement in the future.

182 When Possible, Plan Your Day According to Your Biorhythms

This may be one of those tips that is great in theory but hard to manage in the real world. Keeping a symptom diary (see Chapter 2) can help you to see if there is any kind of pattern to your symptoms. If there is, you can try to schedule your life around that. For example, if you notice that you are more likely to experience diarrhea episodes in the morning, you can try to take the pressure off by avoiding morning appointments. If you are working and notice that there is some predictability as to when your symptoms are at their worst, you may want to talk to your boss about a possible work accommodation or a change in hours.

183 Identify Food Triggers

Food reactivity may contribute to diarrhea episodes. You may find that identifying food sensitivities through the use of an elimination diet or that following the low-FODMAP diet for a while helps to significantly reduce the frequency and intensity of your diarrhea episodes.

184 Use Flushable Wipes. . .

… just don't flush them! Flushable wipes are soft and soothing on the tender tissue of your anus—tissue that can get quite a workout if you have repeated episodes of diarrhea. However, those wipes can be very tough on plumbing. Keep a small can next to your home toilet for disposal.

185 Keep a Toilet Wand Next to Your Toilet for Quick Cleanups

Diarrhea can be messy. These convenient wands can keep your toilet fresh and clean in between your (frequent) trips.

186 Keep Baby Wipes with You for Use When Using Other People's Toilets

I love this tip from Amber J. Tresca, inflammatory bowel disease expert at About.com. If you have a diarrhea episode when in someone else's home, you can wrap a baby wipe around their toilet wand for easy cleanup. If no wand is available, you can try just wiping the toilet down with your baby wipe. In either case, do not flush the wipe! Dispose of it in the trash and then wash your hands thoroughly.

187 Don't Be Afraid to Ask for Help

The unpredictability of IBS diarrhea episodes can be quite disruptive on your life. You may find yourself in situations where you absolutely need to have a backup person; for example, suppose you are a teacher or a parent waiting at a child's bus stop. Don't let embarrassment add to your stress. Pick a trusted person, explain that you experience "stomach problems," and ask them if they can be available to cover for you should you need to make a dash for it.

188 Download a Bathroom Finder App on Your Smartphone

You don't need me to tell you to plan ahead and map out available bathrooms whenever you venture out. Find-a-toilet apps can help you to do just that when you find yourself in an unfamiliar place.

189 It's Okay to Want to Be in Control

The word *control* has gotten a bad rep. All it really means is that you want things to be okay. Your anxiety levels will be lower if you know that you are in control of your ability to get to a bathroom. So when making plans with others, be assertive about what your needs are in terms of what would help you to be more comfortable. Be matter-of-fact about it. You may prefer to take your own car or you may need to check with the driver to ensure that he or she would be willing to make a pit stop should you need one.

Constipation Tips

190 Sleep with a Hot Water Bottle

In addition to using your hot water bottle when you are in pain, try using it to help relax the muscles in your abdomen overnight. This may help your body to feel more ready for a release in the morning.

191 Drink Plenty of Water

Be sure to drink water throughout your day. If your body is not well hydrated, it will react by pulling water from the fecal matter in your intestine. This will result in harder stools that are more difficult to pass. You will know you are drinking enough water if your urine is clear throughout your waking hours (it may be more yellow overnight).

192 Try Bowel Retraining

Bowel retraining is a way of trying to get your intestines to empty in a predictable manner. Here are the steps:

1. Gather a few weeks of data from your symptom diary. This will help you to see if there is any particular time during the day when your body is more likely to be ready to empty. For many people, this is the morning. For others, it is after a large meal.
2. Make it a point to visit the bathroom at a regular time each day, preferably a time based on what you learned from your symptom diary.
3. Before your bathroom visit, eat a large meal or drink a hot beverage (preferably coffee). Both of these can help stimulate intestinal contractions.
4. Get comfortable on the toilet. Bring along some reading material and use your relaxation exercises to calm your body.
5. Without forcing or straining, encourage your body to evacuate.

193 When Your Body Wants to Go, Go!

For some people, lifelong constipation problems develop because of a habit of trying to hold in bowel movements until they get home. Don't be one of these people! If you are feeling urges to evacuate, take yourself to a bathroom and let your body empty. Do not feel embarrassed about this, as that is what bathrooms are for!

Bathroom Accidents

194 Bowel Retraining Can Also Be Helpful for Fecal Incontinence

Sometimes soiling occurs because wet stool from higher up in the colon leaks out around a hard stool mass caused by constipation. In this case, prevention can work as a cure.

195 Keep Yourself as Calm as Possible

If you have not had bathroom accidents in the past, it is most likely that you will not experience them in the future. Although you may protest that you "got there only in the nick of time," the point is that your anal sphincter did hold onto the stool until the appropriate time of release.

196 Remaining Calm Is Particularly Important If You Have Actually Had an Accident in the Past

It is a different story if you have actually soiled yourself in the past. If this occurred in the course of an urgent IBS attack, as opposed to an intestinal illness, you remain at risk for another accident. Most likely this is due to a deficiency in the strength of the anal sphincter muscles. This deficiency may indicate damage to the area due to events such as childbirth, cancer treatment, or anal surgery, or as a result of some other coexisting health condition. Regardless of the cause, keeping your body as calm as possible by using your relaxation exercises and calming self-talk will help quiet the strength of intestinal contractions and allow your sphincter muscles to function to the best of their ability.

197 Be Prepared for Accidents

Preparing ahead of time can help reduce your anxiety, which in turn will help reduce the likelihood of a soiling incident. Adult diapers or feminine hygiene products can bring about great peace of mind. You may also need to keep a change of underwear or clothes with you, just in case.

198 For Road Trips, Think about Investing in a Small, Portable Toilet

You can find various options in camping and marine stores. Portable toilets provide you with a safe, hygienic option if you are somewhere without access to a toilet.

Gas and Bloating Tips

199 Let It Fly!

Everyone passes gas. Holding gas in will increase the pressure inside your colon and may contribute to pain and urgency. If you have the time, it certainly would be more comfortable if you were to go to a private area. However, if you pass gas in public, do not react as if it is the end of the world. It is a natural human function and not something to be ashamed about. As an aside, taking regular yoga classes will surely help desensitize you to passing gas in public. As yoga involves a lot of twisting, it is not unusual for one or more students to audibly pass gas during class. There is even a yoga pose known as "wind-relieving pose!

200 Don't Save Your Bowel Movement for When You Get Home

Here is another reason to go when your body needs to go. A full rectum leaves you at risk for gas retention, leading to uncomfortable bloating. In addition, any passed gas may be more odorous if it has to make its way around a fully formed stool. So, if you feel the urge to have a bowel movement, find the nearest bathroom and let your body evacuate.

201 Think Heat

Your hot water bottle can once again be put to use to help relax intestinal muscles and encourage the passage of trapped gas. In addition, sip on some hot tea. Peppermint tea, in particular, can help relax the muscles lining the intestinal tract, which can help get that gas moving.

202 Get Some Light Exercise

Get your system moving by moving your body. Although vigorous exercise may be too much for your system to handle, gentle exercise such as walking or swimming can be helpful. As mentioned, yoga twists can also help gas to make its way down and out.

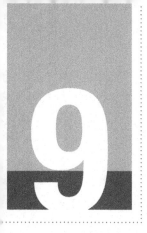

Daily Life

Navigating your way through daily life with IBS can be tricky. Symptoms can be unpredictable, disruptive, and, at times, debilitating. It can be hard to attend to your responsibilities *and* the needs of your body. The following tips will help you to figure out how to best manage your life—including things like work, school, and travel—in spite of your IBS.

Dealing with Unpredictability

203 Mindfulness Can Help You to "Keep It in the Moment"

Remember the saying, "Life is what happens to you when you are making other plans"? Well, IBS can sure find a way to shatter your plans. Mindfulness, the mindset in which you try to focus on what is right in front of you, can help you to develop the flexibility and resilience you will need to deal with unpredicted changes of plans. Mindfulness means just dealing with the way things are going, rather than holding on rigidly to how you think (or want) them to be going.

204 Always Have a Plan B

One way to deal with unpredictability is to be prepared for it. When making future plans, be sure to have a backup plan in case your IBS acts up. This may mean making sure you have phone numbers available should you need to cancel something at the last minute, or making sure you have a way to get home should you need to leave a situation because you're not feeling well.

205 It's Okay to Say "Uncle!" Sometimes

Although you may not want IBS to get the best of you, it is okay to give in to it at times when you are feeling really ill. Continuing to push yourself to remain in a bad situation when your symptoms are severe is the last thing your body needs. It is okay to prioritize what you need to do in order to cope with symptoms, even if that means letting other things go for the time being.

206 Let Your Companions Know That You Are Not Feeling Well

It can be easier to deal with unpredictable symptoms if those around you are keyed in to the fact that you are having a problem. Trying to hide your distress just puts additional stress on your already stressed-out system. When making plans, you can tell others that you may not be able to fully commit as you can't always count on your body to feel well. This will take away some of the pressure of feeling that you need to please others and will allow you to attend to your own needs. You will find more tips for telling others about your condition in Chapter 10.

Work Life

207 Do a Good Job, But Don't Overdo It

Many people who have IBS think that they have to overcompensate for the times when they are ill. This over-compensation can add to one's stress level, and we all know what happens to IBS symptoms when one is stressed. All that is required of you is that you attend to the responsibilities in your job description and that you do your job well. There's no need to be a superhero.

208 Break Any Procrastination Habits

Leaving things to the last minute is not only stressful, but also a pretty risky strategy when you have IBS because you don't know when symptoms might strike. It is much better to get things done when you are feeling well. Some helpful strategies:

1. Break a big task down into manageable pieces.
2. Chunk out time so you can focus solely on one task at a time.
3. Just do it. Don't worry about perfection, just get going.

209 Pay Attention to Your Stress Level

As you go through your workday, pay attention to your overall tension level. If it starts to rise, spend a few minutes engaging in relaxation skills. Think of boxers—they are more effective in the ring if they keep themselves loose and relaxed between punches.

210 If It Feels Safe, Tell Your Boss

If you have a supportive, trustworthy boss, then let her or him know what is going on with your health. This will reduce your anxiety about taking time off or saying no to stressful activities such as travel or public speaking.

211 If Necessary, Go to HR or Utilize EAP Services

If your symptoms are significantly interfering with your work, you may need to engage your company's wellness services. Human resources (HR) may be helpful in letting you know your rights in terms of accommodations and disability benefits. If available, an Employee Assistance Program (EAP) can help with referrals for mental health or legal counseling. If confidentiality is important to you, ask what the policy is regarding information that may be shared with your company's administration.

212 See If You Can Change Your Shift or Work from Home

If your symptoms follow a fairly predictable pattern, you may want to ask your supervisor if you can change your work hours to allow you to be at work when you are more likely to feel well. Alternatively, you may want to ask if you can work from home on days when your symptoms are quite severe.

213 If Necessary, Ask for an Accommodation

IBS is covered under the Americans with Disabilities Act (ADA). This legislation requires employers to make "reasonable accommodations" to assist disabled workers. Modifications can be made to job requirements or work schedules as long as they don't create an "undue hardship" to the employer. To get such an accommodation, all you have to do is ask. Your employer is entitled to require medical documentation regarding your IBS, but must keep the information confidential. If you feel that you have been discriminated against or that your ADA rights have been violated, you can contact the U.S. Equal Employment Opportunity Commission (EEOC).

214 Become Informed about Your Disability Options

Although it typically is better for people's emotional and financial health to be employed, disability may be necessary if you have a severe case of IBS. Your company may offer short-term or long-term disability benefits, or both. The Family and Medical Leave Act (FMLA) entitles you to a certain amount of unpaid leave. For significantly disabling cases of IBS, Social Security Disability Insurance may be an option.

School Life

215 Tell Your Teachers and Other School Administrators about Your IBS

Schools are typically very supportive of students with special needs. Tell your teachers about your IBS if your symptoms will cause you to be absent from school or interfere with your ability to complete assignments on time.

216 If Necessary, Obtain a 504 Plan

Schools that receive federal financial funds must offer a 504 plan to disabled students. A 504 plan spells out what accommodations will be offered to a disabled student so that he or she can enjoy the same educational benefit as a nondisabled student. Reasonable accommodations applicable to IBS include:

1. Access to a nearby bathroom (including a key if necessary) at all times
2. Extended time to complete exams and special projects
3. A modified school schedule
4. Home tutoring if necessary
5. No penalty for lateness, leaving early, or absences

If you feel that you have been discriminated against by your school, you can contact the U.S. Department of Health and Human Services Office for Civil Rights (OCR).

217 Spend Time with Your School Counselor

It might be helpful to form a relationship with your school guidance counselor or school psychologist. These professionals can provide you with support as you try to manage school and a disruptive digestive disorder at the same time. Depending on the counselor, you may be able to use his or her office as a place of refuge when you need to calm your body or your symptoms.

218 Keep Your Body Calm throughout the School Day

Schools are not always relaxing places. Concerns about grades and navigating the ever-changing social scene can cause anxiety. Use calming self-talk, as well as deep breathing and muscle relaxation skills to keep your body as calm as possible as you get through your school day.

219 Enlist the Help of Some Trustworthy Friends. . .

Don't be afraid to tell your friends about your IBS. They can help fill you in on what work you may have missed. This will also help them to be more understanding if you are not up to hanging out or getting something to eat with them.

220 . . .But Be Choosy about Whom You Pick

Unfortunately, school-aged kids are not always the most trustworthy when it comes to personal information. Kids can be flaky and can turn on someone they have previously called a friend if they think it will help their social status. Before letting a friend know about your symptoms, assess whether or not you think they will respect your privacy.

Getting Around

221 Be Prepared before Leaving the House

Having IBS means that those carefree days of "just running out of the house" are a thing of the past. You may need to map out bathroom access (there's an app for that!) or pack a little to-go bag. Here are some things you might want to bring along with you:

- Package of tissues to be used if you are in a toilet that has run out of paper
- Some wet wipes or baby wipes
- Hand sanitizer
- Change of underwear or clothes if you are at risk for soiling

222 Pack Your Own Snacks and Meals

Whether you are going across town or around the world, it might be a good idea to pack foods that you know your body tolerates well. This way you will always have something to eat and can reduce the risk of having to choose foods that will set off your symptoms.

223 Tell the People You Are Traveling With

Let your traveling companions know about any special needs you might have due to your IBS. This may mean the need to avoid certain restaurants or to stop for frequent bathroom breaks.

224 Try Not to Let Your IBS Keep You Trapped at Home

Remember, it is anxiety or foods that can set off symptoms, not geography. Staying calm and eating carefully can help reduce your risk of having to deal with an unhappy GI tract regardless of where you might find yourself. Although home may seem safe, shutting yourself in can contribute to a depressed mood because you are denying yourself the enjoyment of an interesting experience or satisfying social connection. Another way to think about it is that if you are going to have symptoms you might as well have them as you are experiencing something new.

225 When Traveling, Stick as Close to Your Regular Routine as You Can

Changes to your routine can increase your risk of becoming symptomatic. As much as possible, try to stick to your regular eating schedule and sleep–wake cycle.

226 Relieve Stress through Light Exercise

The demands of travel can take a toll on even the healthiest of bodies. Shake off some tension by walking and stretching throughout your day.

227 Stay Hydrated

Air travel, in particular, can be quite dehydrating. When your body becomes dehydrated, it will pull moisture out of your stool, leaving you at risk for constipation. Be sure to drink plenty of water throughout the day.

228 Don't Get Sick

Your digestive tract is already in an unhealthy place. The last thing you need is to wind up with a case of traveler's diarrhea. Be sure to drink only bottled water. Don't eat any foods that seem to have been prepared or stored in an unhygienic manner. Don't eat any raw or undercooked produce, meat, or seafood.

229 Don't Forget to Pack Your Meds

Keep in mind that you may not have the same access to some of your go-to OTC remedies while away from home. Be sure to keep any prescription medications or OTCs in their original packaging.

230 A Portable Toilet May Be Just What You Need for Peace of Mind

As discussed in Chapter 8, a personal Porta Potty is a nice option for long road trips. These types of portable toilets can be quite hygienic and provide an option should you find yourself in an area with no convenient rest stops.

Your Social Life

IBS can wreak havoc with one's social life. For one thing, it is embarrassing to talk about. It is also hard to make plans to spend time enjoying the company of others when you have no idea how your body will be feeling. However, meaningful contact with others is critically important for our overall physical and mental health. Here you will find tips for minimizing the effect that IBS has on your ability to enjoy time spent with other people.

Choosing the Right People

231 Spend Time with Supportive People

IBS is stressful enough—you don't need some toxic person stressing you out even more. Whenever possible, surround yourself with people who are kind, caring, and supportive. That positive energy will be good for your spirits.

232 Whenever Possible, Avoid People Who Are Critical or Unsupportive

It is okay to prioritize your own well-being in this life. Do not feel obliged to spend time with people who are self-centered, critical, or judgmental. Sometimes, this is easier said than done if the unsupportive person is a close relative or coworker. In such cases, you will have to remember that they are the problem, not you. Do not internalize their criticisms or minimization of your distress.

233 Get a Good Sense of the Strengths of Others

In our society, we tend to apply the label of *friend* to the people we bond with and then expect them to have all the wonderful qualities that the word implies. However, people behave based on their personalities, not their labels. You can lessen the disappointment or hurt caused by the actions of others, or in this case, their insensitivity to your IBS, by taking some time to truly assess the personalities of the people in your life. Who can be trusted to keep a secret? Who will help you in a crisis? Who is just fun to hang out with? Match your expectations to the strengths and limitations of others and your relationships will be much more peaceful.

234 Reach Out to Other People Who Have IBS

The Internet has been one of the best things to happen for people who have IBS. Online support groups allow you to connect and speak openly with others about the symptoms and challenges you are dealing with. The Irritable Bowel Syndrome Self Help and Support Group (http://www.ibsgroup.org/) is a wonderful online forum. You may also find support groups on Facebook.

Telling Others

235 Telling Others Can Significantly Cut Down on Anxiety

It can be very stressful to try to hide something as disruptive as IBS from others. You will find yourself trying to make excuses and then having to remember to keep your lies straight. You will take a great load off of your shoulders (and your colon!) if you are up-front with others about what you are dealing with.

236 Don't Be Ashamed

Yes, symptoms are embarrassing, but they are not a reflection of your character. They are merely a sign that something is wrong with your digestive tract. You will be more comfortable talking to others about your IBS if you do not view it as a personal failing.

237 Develop a Matter-of-Fact Attitude

Digestive symptoms are just that, symptoms. They are simply responses that our bodies have—no different than sneezing. If you speak openly and calmly about your symptoms, in a matter-of-fact manner, you will take a lot of the awkwardness out of the conversation.

238 Everyone Experiences Digestive Symptoms

One way to help yourself feel more comfortable telling others about your IBS is to remember that everyone has a large intestine! Therefore, at one point or another, everyone has had similar symptoms to the ones you are dealing with. The only difference is that you are dealing with them on a chronic basis. Since no one likes to experience digestive symptoms, most people will be empathic.

239 They May Have IBS, Too

It is estimated that 15 to 20 percent of the population has IBS. Thus, the odds are fairly high that if you tell someone you have IBS, that person is very likely to say that he or she does, too!

240 Start with Trustworthy Individuals

It's okay to start off easy if you are new to telling others about your IBS. Pick people that you know will be supportive and can be trusted to keep the information to themselves.

241 Don't Tell Untrustworthy Individuals

Unless you are very comfortable with having others know your personal business, choose your confidants wisely. In other words, maybe you don't want to tell the town gossip. Similarly, if you are a teenager at risk for some "mean girl" bullying, be careful which friends you tell. Another situation in which you might want to be extra cautious is at work. Although by law you can't be discriminated against because of your IBS, not all workplaces are law abiding.

242 Don't Let the Turkeys Get You Down

Some people are limited in their ability to be empathic. Suppose you tell someone who turns out to be unsupportive or minimizes your distress. Take this as information: you have just learned something about this person's trustworthiness. Don't go back to the empty well. Let this one go and focus your efforts on people who are truly caring.

243 Inform Others on a Need-to-Know Basis

You don't have to tell everyone about your IBS, of course. The most important consideration is whether it is in your best interest to let them know about your distress. If it will make your life easier, then tell. If telling certain people will complicate your life or cause you more stress, then feel free to keep it to yourself.

244 Time It Well

Timing in life is everything. Don't tell others when they are rushing out the door or engrossed in a television show. You may also want to get to know a person well before sharing your health history. Timing becomes a significantly important issue when on the dating scene.

245 Avoid TMI (Too Much Information)!

When telling others about your IBS, there is no need to go into graphic detail. Keep it simple; for example, "I have IBS, which means that I have chronic digestive symptoms."

246 Tell Others What Your Needs Are

Be open about how IBS affects your life and how it can affect your interactions with others. Let people know if you need to be near a bathroom at all times or that you are prone to canceling plans at the last minute. Be clear about your dietary needs; for example, "I am on a special diet for my stomach and I need to be careful about what foods I eat."

247 Be Gracious in the Face of Unwanted Advice

Some people believe that they are experts in everything and would love to tell you what you should do to make your IBS all better. Try to see through to the underlying motivation, which is to be of help. You can say something like, "Thank you for your advice. It is nice of you to want to help, but at this point, I have a pretty good idea of what is going to help me and what is going to make things worse for me."

Social Outings

248 Eat Lightly before You Go

Many people with IBS make the mistake of avoiding foods altogether before a social outing. Keep in mind that your digestive tract will hum along more smoothly if it is given food on a consistent basis. Eating before you go also keeps you from being too hungry and thus being at risk for eating foods that you know that you don't tolerate well.

249 Tell Your Host or Hostess of Any Special Food Needs

There is a growing awareness of the reality of food allergies and sensitivities. Before attending an event centered around food, it might be a good idea to contact the hosts to let them know about your dietary needs. This way you can find out if there will be any appropriate options for you or if you need to bring your own food. Warning the hosts ahead of time should also save you from having food pressed on you. And, if the hosts know what you can and cannot eat, you will not be hurting their feelings if you choose not to eat the food they have prepared.

250 Cope with Any Anticipatory Anxiety

Anticipatory anxiety is the anxiety that one experiences before arriving at a new situation. It is triggered by an underlying fear of the unknown. Generally, anticipatory anxiety goes away as soon as you enter into the feared situation. You can work to keep yourself as calm as possible before the time of your social outing by keeping your to-do list light and actively engaging in relaxation exercises.

251 Cope with Any Social Anxiety

Social anxiety is a form of extreme self-consciousness that causes a person to experience anxiety symptoms when interacting with others. Having IBS alongside social anxiety is quite a double whammy, as fears of being embarrassed by one's digestive symptoms are heightened. Try to remember that most people are too busy thinking about their own social performance to be judging you! Use relaxation exercises to keep yourself calm. You can also take breaks from the social occasion as needed to keep your baseline anxiety level lower. If your social anxiety is quite severe, and does seem to aggravate your IBS, you may want to consider getting treatment for it. Antidepressant medications and cognitive behavioral therapy (CBT) are two effective choices.

252 Devise a Comfortable Exit Strategy

It can bring great peace of mind, and therefore calm your body, if you know that you have a good exit plan. This may mean taking your own car or letting those you traveled with know that you may need to leave before the event is finished.

253 Choose Your Food and Drinks Carefully

While out in public, be sure to only eat foods that you know your body can tolerate well. Don't let the fear of offending another person get in the way of prioritizing your own self-care. Remember that alcohol can be an irritant, so drink minimally.

254 Distract Yourself from Body Sensations

When a person has been traumatized, he or she is at risk for developing hypervigilance. This is an attempt by the brain to scan the environment for cues associated with the trauma. Such hypervigilance can develop in a person who has IBS. You yourself may find that you have become very in tune with inner body sensations that you fear may be a sign that an IBS attack is imminent. Try to remember that not every twinge or cramp is a sign of trouble. Take some deep breaths and distract yourself by focusing on the events and people surrounding you.

255 Enjoy The Distraction

You may need to push yourself to get away from the comfort of your own home, but you may be glad that you did. Interacting with others—finding out what they have been up to, sharing laughs and old memories, and making new memories—can be great for your mood and serve to distract you from your digestive distress.

Restaurants

256 Check the Menu Ahead of Time

Many restaurants publish their menus online. This allows you to look at a menu to ensure that the restaurant has options that are appropriate for you. If necessary, you can call ahead to find out what dietary accommodations can be made.

257 Tell Your Dining Companions

You will feel much more comfortable if you tell the people that you are dining with that you have a digestive health condition. You may need to tell others that a certain restaurant will not work for you because it lacks appropriate menu options. Your companions may also need to be prepared should you need to leave early or just spend extra time in the bathroom.

258 Have a Comfortable Exit Plan

Just knowing that you can get up and walk out can help relieve any gut-wrenching anxiety. You are not trapped in a restaurant simply because you have placed a food order. Your only responsibility is to pay for the food! If you need to leave because you are feeling quite ill, inform your companions, leave enough money to cover the cost of your meal, and go.

259 Use Relaxation Exercises

Of course, the goal is to enjoy your meal out, not to get up and leave. Improve your chances of having a calm system by using deep breathing and calming self-talk skills to keep your anxiety low.

260 Order Smart

Restaurants can be filled with potential landmines for a person with IBS. Be careful about your food choices. Keep your portion sizes small. Avoid eating anything that is creamy, greasy, or deep-fried. And don't forget that excess alcohol can be a digestive system irritant, as well as serve to cloud your judgment regarding food choices.

Your Dating Life

261 Pick the Time to Tell

Something as personal as your digestive health is not something that you need to share on your first date. View the first date a bit like a job interview—you are collecting information about the other person. Once it seems as if a new love prospect might become a sure thing, you can tell them about your IBS.

262 Be Open about Your Needs

Let your date know what your needs are, whether that involves eating certain foods or not traveling far from home. Clear communication can serve not only to avoid the stress of secrecy but also to deepen your sense of connection to the other person.

263 Know Your Strengths

The person you are dating has chosen to spend time with you because he or she likes you for what you are. Keep in mind all of the things that make you wonderful. This will help overcome your brain's tendency to make a big deal out of your IBS.

264 Assess the Strengths of the Other Person

A common dating mistake is to be so focused on trying to make a good impression on the other person that you lose sight of the fact that you should also be deciding if that person is good for you. Take an inventory. Does this person have the qualities you desire in a mate? Is he or she caring, trustworthy, supportive? Are there any signs of a major mood disorder, personality disorder, or substance abuse problem? For a relationship to be successful, you need to be comfortable and satisfied with the other person.

265 It's Okay to Lean on Someone Else

Sometimes we all try too hard to be strong and independent. We are not islands, but are part of a social species. It is okay to ask your date to assist you in whatever way she or he can with your IBS. Let your date do the research regarding restaurants and restrooms. See if she or he has some ideas for passing the time enjoyably even if you need to stay in. Perhaps your date would be willing to accompany you to doctors' appointments to be a second set of ears. If so, it would be a good sign of your date's overall character.

266 Break It Off if Your Needs Are Not Being Met

Every one of my single patients has heard my expert advice on dating: "Run!" If the person that you are dating cannot handle your IBS, then he or she is not the person for you. Everyone deserves a partner in life who has the capacity to join together to deal with the challenges that life brings. If you lose a relationship because of your special needs, it was not really a quality relationship. Look at it as if you dodged a bullet.

Your Sex Life

267 Keep The Lines of Communication Open

Sexual relationships can be challenging to navigate even when both individuals are healthy. An unpredictable digestive disorder like IBS can prove to be quite a challenge for the individuals involved to manage. The best thing you can do is to be very open about where you are—mentally and physically—in regard to your intimate life, and very open to listening to your partner's needs and concerns. Physical intimacy is just a part of overall intimacy. Deep sharing can truly connect people even if their bodies are not cooperating.

268 It's Okay to Say No

It may be near-impossible to enjoy yourself sexually if you are in pain or discomfort. Don't be afraid to tell your partner if you are not up for physical intimacy.

269 Don't Lose Sight of the Other Person's Needs

Just as it is important to be open with your partner about where you are at sexually, it is also essential that you take the time to listen to your partner's thoughts and feelings about your intimate life. The worst thing to do is to ignore the whole subject because you are not up to having sex. Let your partner know that you are aware of his or her needs and that you will do your best to be a sexual partner on the days when you feel well.

270 Seek Counseling if Necessary

You may find that trying to figure out how to have a satisfying sexual relationship is too much to handle given the limitations that IBS (and perhaps other coexisting health problems) imposes on your body. If this is the case, consulting with a qualified professional may be very helpful.

Family Life

Like many health conditions, IBS doesn't just affect those who have it; it also affects the people who love them. The stress of dealing with IBS can strain a marriage, interfere with one's ability to be a parent, and have an impact on siblings. In this chapter, we will look at ways to minimize the impact that IBS has on your family life, as well as some helpful tips for dealing with a child's IBS.

Marriage

271 ## The More Support You Get from Your Spouse, the Better You Will Feel

Research has shown that people with IBS who have supportive spouses have better treatment outcomes than those who have unsupportive spouses. Lower levels of marital conflict are also associated with a better response to IBS management strategies. If your spouse is unsupportive, or your relationship is marked by too much conflict, discuss your concerns with your spouse to see if he or she will come on board as a more helpful partner.

272 ## Don't be Afraid to Speak Up and Share Your Own Thoughts on How Best to Manage Your Symptoms

Sometimes a well-meaning spouse may try to take control of your IBS. Let her or him know that you appreciate the help, but share the fact that research suggests that IBS patients do much better when they perceive that they are in control of their own health. This means that you ask your spouse to follow your lead in terms of which doctors to see, which remedies to try, what foods to eat, and the like.

273 ## Spell Out What You Can Handle and What Your Spouse Will Handle

The clearer the communication in a marriage, the smoother things will run. Spell out which aspects of IBS you need help with and which aspects you can manage on your own.

274 Ignore the Unhelpful

Out of ignorance or frustration, your spouse (and other people!) may share unhelpful advice with you. Sometimes this can take the form of blaming, in which they tell you that you are eating the wrong foods or that you are just too stressed. In these cases, you can thank them for their concern without getting into why their advice won't work for you.

275 Express Gratitude and Empathy

Let your spouse know how much you appreciate his or her support. Be sure to thank your spouse when he or she takes over responsibilities that IBS prevents you from attending to. Don't forget to acknowledge the fact that IBS affects your spouse's life as well, but do this without self-blame. Neither of you asked for this—it is a reality in your life, but it is no one's fault.

276 Don't Overlook the Physical Aspect of Your Relationship

As discussed in Chapter 10, a chronic health problem like IBS can have a significant negative impact on a couple's sex life. It is neither healthy nor enjoyable to force yourself to do anything that you don't want to do because you don't feel up to it. However, it is important to maintain open communication with your spouse on the subject, so that he or she knows that these needs are not being totally overlooked by you.

277 Marital Counseling May Help Shore Up Your Relationship against the Stress of IBS

If your efforts at improving communication and reducing conflict are unsuccessful, you may want to consider marriage counseling. Meeting with a qualified professional can help the two of you to better meet the challenges that a chronic health problem like IBS brings into a marriage.

Being a Parent

278 It's Okay to Prioritize Your Own Needs over Other People's Wants

With IBS, there will be times when you will need to take care of the needs and demands of your body. This may mean that your children will have to wait until you have done so before you can attend to their desires. Try not to feel guilty about this. The better you take care of yourself, the better able you will be to take care of them.

279 When Possible, Have Backup Help

If your symptoms are interfering with your ability to meet the *needs* of your children, you may have to ask other people to help out. This may mean that you have to hire a babysitter or ask a family member to assist you if you have small children who cannot be left unattended while you are in the bathroom. Similarly, you may have a friend who is willing to take over if you cannot wait with your children at the bus stop or pick them up from school.

280 Cook the Foods You Need to Eat

Don't force yourself to eat foods that you know your body doesn't handle well. You can round out the meal by preparing some items that are appealing to all and some items that you can eat without aggravating your symptoms.

281 Explain Your IBS to Your Children at a Level They Can Understand

Trying to hide your IBS from your children is an added stress that your body does not need to deal with. How much you tell them will depend on their ages and personalities. If they are quite young, you can just say that your belly hurts sometimes. If they are school-aged, they will be able to understand some of the science behind IBS. If they are worriers, assure them that IBS is challenging but not life-threatening.

When Your Child Has IBS

282 Work Closely with Your Child's Doctors to Establish a Management Plan

Whenever possible, work with a doctor that both you and your child are comfortable with. Express any concerns about your child's symptoms and diagnosis. Seek a second opinion if you feel that the doctor is not addressing your concerns adequately. Before trying any new dietary approach, be sure to get clearance from your child's doctor to ensure that your child will be getting adequate nutrition.

283 Talk to Your Child about How Digestion Works and What May Be Going Wrong

For small children, you can find a picture book on digestion that shows them what is going on inside their bodies. Older children may have been exposed to this information in school. At a level that the child can understand, you can explain what might be going wrong and what she or he can do to help make things better.

284 Teach Ways to Self-Soothe the Pain

These strategies will also be age dependent. Small children may choose to hug a stuffed animal, while older children may find it more comfortable to listen to music. Guided imagery (see Chapter 8) can be very effective with children. Regardless of your child's age, he or she can use the power of imagination to envision what the pain looks like and what would be needed for the pain to go away.

285 Work with Your Child to Be More Matter-of-Fact about Bowel Movements

Assure your child that going to the bathroom is a regular part of life for everyone. If your child is more likely to be constipated, work together to establish a regular time for bathroom trips. Make it a fun and special time with you. If your child has had to deal with urgent diarrhea, work together to use relaxation exercises to keep her or him from panicking and making things worse.

286 Let the School Know

Your child may be quite anxious about trying to meet the demands of school while dealing with the demands of his or her body. Let the school know what is going on with your child. If necessary, ask for a 504 plan. As discussed in Chapter 9, a 504 plan spells out any special accommodations that your child may need, such as bathroom access, additional time to complete assignments, or modified class schedules.

287 Consider Bringing Your Child to a Qualified Therapist

As discussed in Chapter 4, two forms of psychotherapy have research support for reducing IBS symptoms. There is a lot of evidence that hypnotherapy is effective in helping children who experience chronic bellyaches. Cognitive behavioral therapy (CBT) is a good option if your child is experiencing a lot of anxiety about having IBS.

288 Don't Make It All about the IBS

Although you don't want to minimize your child's distress, you don't want to dwell on it either. Try to keep family routines as normal as possible and do what you can to ensure that your child's life is as well-balanced as it can be.

289 Balance Out the Needs of All Family Members

Trying to meet the needs of all children in a family is one of the hardest parts of parenting. Although the child with IBS will need some extra attention, work to make sure that other children do not get resentful. You may need to allow time for siblings to vent their feelings to you. Siblings are less resentful if they feel they are part of the solution. Ask them for their ideas on how to accommodate the sick child while still having fun as a family.

Stress Management

The link between stress and the digestive system is deep and complex. The stress of modern life, as well as that associated with having IBS, can serve to worsen your symptoms. Luckily, there are things you can do to calm your body and your mind to help reduce the effects of daily stressors on your IBS.

The Stress Response

290 Our Body's Stress Response Developed as a Way to Keep Us Alive in the Face of Predators

When we were evolving as a species, our bodies developed a fight or flight response to perceived threats. This stress response triggered a variety of changes, all designed to help us to either fight or flee any hungry lions we may have encountered. Some of these changes involve the digestive system, because when we were faced with a hungry predator, it was more important to stay alive than to digest our lunch. In today's world, our stress triggers are not quite as dramatic as hungry predators, but they tend to be a lot more frequent.

291 The Stress Response Can Trigger a Variety of Symptoms

When our stress response kicks in, the following body changes occur:

- Heart rate increases
- Breathing speeds up
- Muscles tense
- Stomach emptying slows
- Colon contractions speed up
- Bladder muscles relax

292 The Effects of Stress Can Be Offset by Stress Management Activities

Stress management activities are things that we can do to either turn off the stress response or help our bodies to be more resilient in the face of modern-day challenges. These activities have been shown to have a calming effect on the central nervous system. And due to the brain-gut connection, anything that calms your nervous system is going to have a beneficial effect on the functioning of your digestive system.

Relaxation Exercises

293 Relaxation Exercises Can Help Turn Off the Body's Flight-or-Fight Reflex

Relaxation exercises include visualization, deep breathing techniques, and muscle relaxation exercises. Regular practice of these techniques can lower your body's baseline anxiety level and help you to actively calm your body during times of high stress. You can use these exercises during an IBS attack to help calm your system and ease your pain.

294 Visualization Can Be Used for Calming

Visualization is a technique that you can use to calm your mind and distract it from the "what if" kinds of thoughts that raise anxiety. One calming visualization technique is to close your eyes and imagine that you are in a place that represents beauty and safety for you. It can be a real place or somewhere in your imagination. Use all of your senses to firmly ground you in that place; in other words, imagine what you see, smell, hear, taste, and feel.

295 Visualization Can Also Be Used to Promote Healing

As discussed in Chapter 8, a visualization technique called guided imagery can be used to encourage your body to move back toward a state of health. While closing your eyes, allow an image to form of the body part that is giving you the most pain or trouble. Don't censor the image, just work with what comes up. Then gently manipulate the image so that it moves toward a healthier one. For example, if you were to visualize your bowels as being in a twisted knot, imagine gently massaging them so that the knot loosens.

296 Deep Breathing Techniques Can Be Used Anytime, Anywhere

As part of the body's stress response, breathing becomes rapid and shallow. Taking slow, deep breaths using your diaphragm can help turn off the stress response and help your body to relax. Like all skills, you will get better at using breathing techniques with practice. Once you are proficient, you can actively slow your breathing anytime you feel yourself getting anxious.

297 It May Take a Little Practice to Develop Your Ability to Breathe Deeply

The first step is to find your diaphragm. Place one of your hands on your belly right above your belly button. Feel how this part of your body rises and falls as you breathe. Keep your chest and shoulder muscles relaxed. Let your body breathe by itself—don't work too hard. As you get more in touch with this deep method of breathing, try to slow your breath down so that you are inhaling to the count of three and exhaling to the count of three.

298 Progressive Muscle Relaxation (PMR) Can Help Ease Muscle Tension

If you have ever watched a professional boxing match, you know that the boxers dance in between punches. This is to keep their muscles as loose as possible while saving up their energy to deliver the most powerful blows. In sharp contrast to boxers, many of us walk around all day with excessive muscle tension, draining us of energy and keeping us on alert, with the result that our stress response is chronically activated. Progressive muscle relaxation exercises are a way to learn to let go of this unnecessary muscle tension.

299 PMR Is Not Hard to Learn

Sit in a quiet place, imagine yourself in your peaceful space, and slow down your breathing. Starting at the top of your head, pick a muscle group and tense it to the count of three as you inhale, then relax those muscles as you exhale. For example, scrunch up your forehead muscles and then smooth them out. Work your way down your body, one muscle group at a time. Focus on the different sensations you feel with a tense muscle versus a relaxed muscle. Feel your body growing looser, warmer, and heavier, as feelings of relaxation make their way down your body.

300 Moving Meditations Can Have a Calming Effect on the Body

As discussed in Chapter 4, the ancient moving meditation practices of yoga and tai chi have been shown to have a very calming effect on your nervous system. With regular practice, you will experience a lowered baseline anxiety level, elevation of mood, and reduced reactivity to normal life stressors. All of this calming will be very soothing to your digestive tract and help to offset the role that stress is playing in exacerbating your symptoms.

301 Spend Some Time Outdoors

Whether you call it vitamin N (Nature) or "green exercise," spending time outside can have an extremely beneficial effect on your overall health as well as being great for reducing stress. Go outside on your lunch break, take a walk around the block each day, or spend some time gardening. (As you will see in Chapter 13, gardening may offer an additional benefit of exposing you to some healthy bacteria!)

Healthy Thinking

302 What We Think Can Very Much Affect How We Feel, Both Physically and Emotionally

Due to the close connection between the brain and the gut, anxious thoughts can trigger or exacerbate IBS symptoms. The problem is that when you have been traumatized by stressful symptoms, it is only natural to be anxious about future symptoms. In a classic chicken-and-egg scenario, this anxiety then serves to increase the risk of actually experiencing the very symptoms you were afraid of. Luckily, you can actively work to challenge and replace these anxious thoughts.

303 Watch Out for the "Uh-Oh"

A common aftereffect of a traumatic event is to become hypervigilant. This means that a person continually scans the environment for signs that the feared event will reoccur. You may note this in yourself as you are constantly paying attention to inner signals of digestive distress. In response to any kind of cramp, pain, or gas bubble, you may think, "Uh-oh, here comes trouble." However, with IBS, this "uh-oh" thought might be enough, all by itself, to set off symptoms. You can work to be calmer in reaction to inner sensations by telling yourself that not every inner twinge means that a full-blown attack is coming on. Do some deep breathing, distract your mind, and see what happens.

304 Watch Out for Those "What If . . . ?" Thoughts

When our brains hit us with "what if . . . ?" scenarios, we experience anxiety related to that future event, even though it is not happening to us right now. An example would be "What if I get to the party and my IBS starts to act up?" The problem with these anxiety-based future projections is that they focus on the problem, without offering any kind of solution.

305 Swap Out "What If . . . ?" for "What Would I Do If . . . ?"

A better strategy is to identify reality-based concerns and then come up with a plan. So, sticking with our example, you would say to yourself, "Yes, it's possible that I could experience symptoms while I'm at the party, but I don't know that for sure. I will make sure to bring my own car, so that I know I can leave if I don't feel well."

306 Keep It in the Moment

Mindfulness is an attempt to keep your focus on what is going on in the here and now. This means to work actively to distract yourself from future worries and past memories and deal with how your body is feeling right here, right now. You will find more tips for cultivating mindfulness later in this chapter.

307 Don't "Awfulize"

When we think to ourselves "This is horrible," our bodies react as if whatever is going on is the very worst thing that could happen. Your body might be feeling pretty lousy, and perhaps at a very inconvenient time, but quantifying the experience as the worst thing that could happen sets off alarm bells in your system. These alarm bells trigger the body's stress response, which can then make your symptoms worse.

308 Use Calming Self-Talk

When you feel anxious, calming self-talk can be helpful. For example, you might tell yourself, "Yes, this is pretty bad right now, but I can get through it. Let me work to calm myself and see if that helps my system to settle." Anything you can do to quiet your body instead of agitating it will only help.

309 Other People Will Not Judge You Based on Your IBS

People will not think less of you because you go to the bathroom a lot. Bathroom visits and digestive symptoms are something that everyone experiences, not just people who have IBS. People who like you like you because you are you. They will not think poorly of you just because you have digestive problems.

310 Don't Make the Mistake of Assuming That Geography Causes Symptoms

IBS has the potential to cause a person to become quite isolated, particularly if he or she decides to avoid going out so as to avoid being sick. Sure, you might be more comfortable being home if symptoms strike, but it is anxiety that triggers symptoms, not the particular situation in which you find yourself. Anxiety is something you can gain better control of, through the use of relaxation strategies and calming self-talk. Get better at keeping your anxiety level low (and watching out for dietary triggers!) and you may find that your body becomes more trustworthy.

311 Talk to Yourself as If You Were Your Own Child

Many of us have an inner self-critic. This negative voice might engage in a lot of trash talk, but you don't have to pay attention. You are not well—you deserve to be nurtured and loved, not criticized and punished. Speak to yourself the way you would if you were trying to soothe a sick or frightened child. Be kind and nonjudgmental.

312 Don't Keep Questioning Your Diagnosis

Research has found that if basic diagnostic testing shows no signs of another disease and you have none of the red-flag symptoms discussed in Chapter 1, then most likely your diagnosis of IBS is an accurate one. Therefore, try not to let your thoughts run away from you, leading you to fear that you have cancer or some other life-threatening illness. Remind yourself that your IBS is just acting up, and hold on until symptoms ease.

313 Look for the Silver Lining

The old adage that every dark cloud has a silver lining is a wise one. Although having IBS is a rotten thing, there may be some ways in which it has been helpful. Perhaps it has prompted you to work less, take better care of yourself, or eat healthier foods. This more balanced perspective can help you to better cope on days when things seem bleak.

Self-Esteem

314 Remember, You Are Not Your IBS

Because of the embarrassing nature of its symptoms, IBS is often experienced differently by the person who has it than other health problems. Often, those with IBS experience unnecessary shame that then takes a toll on their self-esteem. It is important to remember that IBS is something that has happened to you—you did not cause it and you don't have to be defined by it.

315 Make a List of All of Your Positive Qualities

Our minds tend to minimize our successful experiences and magnify our limitations. For example, you may forget a compliment minutes after hearing one but remember a criticism 20 years later! To compensate for this, it is helpful to sit down and make a list of all of your strengths, talents, and assets. If this is really difficult for you, ask someone who knows you well to help you. Having a concrete list of all of the things that make you special and wonderful can help offset your feelings of shame related to your IBS.

316 See Yourself as Others See You

Another mental tendency is to be much more judgmental when it comes to ourselves than others. We tend to focus on every little detail about ourselves. However, with others, we tend to have broader views. Rather than defining yourself as a person who is difficult because IBS affects what you can do and what you can eat, work to see yourself the way that others see you. Other people may or may not know that you have IBS, but they value you for qualities that have nothing to do with the state of your digestive health.

317 There's No Need to Work Harder to Make Up for Your IBS

Many people who have IBS tend to push themselves to be overly productive to make up for the times when their symptoms interfere with their ability to function and attend to responsibilities. However, doing so puts unnecessary stress on both your nervous system and your digestive tract and may exacerbate your symptoms. When you are feeling well, put in a good day's work, but remember to pace yourself and to be alert to your body's signals that you are putting too much pressure on yourself.

318 Be Nurturing to Yourself by Allowing Yourself to Take Sick Time-Outs

When your symptoms are chronic, it can be hard to know when to give in to them. Sometimes, you just need a little time for your system to settle down and then you can continue on with your day. At other times, you may need to run up the white flag and make tending to yourself your number one priority. When in doubt, ask yourself what you would advise your best friend to do. Often we are much more nurturing of others than we are of ourselves.

Mindfulness

319 Mindfulness Practice Is a Way to Help Keep Your Mind in the Moment

Mindfulness practices are things that you do to help you to stay aware of the present moment. Such practices can help reduce anxiety, making it less likely that you will be stirred up by future fears.

320 Learn What Mindfulness Feels Like by Eating a Piece of Dark Chocolate

There is a classic mindfulness exercise that involves eating a raisin, but since raisins are high in FODMAPs, a better choice is a piece of quality dark chocolate. Before putting the chocolate in your mouth, spend a few moments examining its shape and color. Bring it to your nose and smell it. Put a small piece in your mouth and pay attention to how it tastes. Does it taste different depending on which part of your tongue it is on? Pay attention to the sensations that occur as the chocolate melts and makes its way down your throat. Do all of this in an unhurried way, focusing strongly on the sensations that you experience in the here and now.

321 Expand Your Mindfulness Practice to Some of Your Daily Routines

Set your intention to use the same focus on the sensations in the here and now as you go through some of the ordinary tasks of your day. Work on being mindful while in the shower, brushing your teeth, or preparing dinner. You will certainly enjoy your meals more if you actually pay attention while eating them!

322 Set a Timer on Your Smartphone to Orient You Back to the Present

Some people find it helpful to have their smartphone chirp at regular intervals to remind them to bring their awareness to the present. You can pick whatever interval works for you. When you hear the timer go off, pay attention to what it is that you are doing right then, in that moment.

323 Add Sitting Meditation to Your Regular Routine

Sitting meditation, as discussed in Chapter 4, is a wonderful complement to a mindfulness practice. During a sitting meditation you are practicing the skill of being focused on the present as you keep bringing your attention back to your breath. This practice will enhance your ability to be more aware of the present as you make your way through your day.

Financial Stress

324 Put Your Budget on Paper

Often worries, such as those about money, just bang around in our heads, causing stress to the whole system. Put some time aside to make a budget for yourself. This will help you to identify where the financial problems lie. Are you spending more than you are taking in? Are you paying high interest on debt? With this information you can start to brainstorm solutions—figuring out what steps you can take to try to find some financial stability.

325 Remember to Keep It in the Day

Remember to differentiate between reality-based concerns and "what if"–type fears. You may be fearful that at some point you will have to declare bankruptcy or that your home will go into foreclosure. Figure out what you can do today to address those concerns and then bring your awareness to the fact that those things are not happening today. You will figure out a way to deal with those scary things when the situation is right there in front of you. The old adage "you can't build a bridge until you get to the river" can be very helpful for these anxious projections.

326 Have Regularly Scheduled Budget Meetings with Yourself or Your Significant Other

Businesses do not spend every moment focused on their finances—if they did they would never get anything done! Set aside a time, either weekly or biweekly, to pay your bills and go over your finances. Once that is done, do your best to not think about money until the next regularly scheduled meeting.

327 Let Go of Shame

It is very human to be very hard on yourself, particularly when it comes to being in financial straits. If your money problems are due to overspending, then shift from shame to regret and learn from your mistakes. However, often money problems happen even when people are trying to be responsible. Let go of unnecessary shame and negative self-talk and just deal with the problems at hand.

328 Seek Help

Unless you were a finance major in college, it is likely that you have been given very little guidance as to how to manage money. Read books or take classes to learn better financial management skills. If necessary, seek the professional help of a financial advisor or debt counselor.

Self-Care
Strategies

Modern life is busy. Often we are so caught up in tending to all of our responsibilities that caring for our bodies ends up low on our lists. However, the intensity of IBS symptoms forces you to pay attention to the needs of your body. You can find the silver lining in the dark cloud that is IBS by using your digestive distress as a prompt for better self-care.

Healthy Gut Bacteria

329 **The Health of Your Gut Bacteria Can Have a Significant Effect on Your Symptoms**

As discussed in Chapter 1, scientists are focusing in on the role that gut bacteria play in the development of IBS and other digestive and nondigestive chronic disorders. Our intestines are populated by countless strains of bacteria, yeast, and other microorganisms. These organisms are known collectively as your microflora, and this inner world is called your microbiome. As part of your self-care regimen, don't neglect this world that teems within you.

330 **Whenever Possible, Avoid Antibiotics**

Antibiotics can wreak havoc on the balance of your gut bacteria and are not effective against viruses—save them for clear-cut bacterial infections. This tip does not apply to the specific antibiotics prescribed for SIBO. Those antibiotics act on bacteria within the small intestine, not the large intestine.

331 **Gut Bacteria Are Affected by Stress, so Be Sure to Engage in Activities That Counteract the Stress in Your Life**

Research has shown that both acute and chronic stress can cause a change in the balance of your gut bacteria. Try to add the stress management activities that we covered in Chapter 12 to your regular routine.

332 **Take in Friendly Bacteria**

As discussed in Chapter 4, it is possible to improve the health of your microbiome through the use of probiotics. These can be in the form of probiotic supplements or fermented foods.

When buying a probiotic supplement, make sure that you are buying a product with live strains that are guaranteed to be alive at the time of use. Fermented vegetables, yogurt, kefir, and kombucha are all excellent probiotic-containing fermented food options.

333 Decrease Your Intake of Refined Sugar and Processed Foods

Consuming high levels of simple carbohydrates, through excess sugar and refined grains, is thought to contribute to gut dysbiosis, which is another name for microbial imbalance. To increase the health of your gut flora, eat whole foods—lean protein, vegetables, fruits, and healthy fats.

334 Digging in the Dirt May Be Beneficial for Your Microbiome

The so-called hygiene hypothesis suggests that excessive hygiene practices are one of the reasons behind rising rates of immune system disorders. It is thought that interacting with dirt, through gardening or outside play, exposes people to microorganisms that may be helpful to the gut. Gardening has an added benefit: growing your own organic vegetables and fruits will provide you with optimal nutrition—great for your gut bacteria and your overall health!

Physical Exercise

335 Physical Exercise May Be Challenging, but It Is a Great Stress Reducer

IBS pain or diarrhea urgency may make it hard to exercise. However, through brainstorming and some planning you can find a way to move your body in spite of your symptoms.

336 Write Your Exercise Schedule in Your Day Planner

You will be more likely to meet your exercise goals if you schedule exercise into your daily routine. View it as you would a job or a doctor's appointment and show up at the allotted time. Although it can be hard to get started, focus on how well you will feel when you are done.

337 Have Your Exercise Clothes Readily Available

You will be less likely to find an excuse not to exercise if you have readied your exercise clothes ahead of time. This may mean that you have them right alongside your bed for a morning exercise session or packed in a bag in your car so that you can hit the gym after work.

338 Choose a Low-Impact Option if Intense Exercise Results in Runner's Diarrhea

Your body will still benefit from the movement and muscle-toning effects of the following activities, even if it can't handle more strenuous, cardio-type exercise:

- Dancing
- Swimming
- Walking
- Weight training
- Yoga

339 Avoid Eating Two Hours before Exercising

Try to schedule your exercise during a time when your digestive system is not actively digesting your last meal. This will help it to stay quieter as you work out.

340 Avoid Eating and Drinking Things That Have the Potential for Strengthening Intestinal Contractions before Your Workouts

In the time leading up to your planned exercise, avoid:

- Hot drinks
- Caffeine-containing drinks
- Fatty foods
- Gassy foods

341 Explore Exercise-at-Home Options

If your IBS symptoms prevent you from getting to the gym or exercising outside, you may find that home exercise is a better fit for you. The biggest challenge to a home exercise routine is discipline!

342 Exercise Videos Are a Great Way to Keep It Interesting

If you are a person who gets bored easily, exercise videos may be a great option. Many are available for free or for purchase online. Your public library may be another great resource for borrowing free videos. With videos, you can change up the pace and the activity whenever you like—all within the comfort of your own home.

343 Video Game Consoles Are a Great Way to Make It Fun

Manufacturers of video games have jumped onto the exercise bandwagon. Games are now available that encourage you to move, stretch, and strengthen your body. Whether you play the games by yourself or increase your motivation by playing with a partner, the game aspect will help keep your motivation up.

344 Make Space

You can affirm your intention to make physical exercise a regular part of your life if you set aside space in your home to exercise comfortably. You may want to set up a dedicated corner for your yoga mat or make sure you can move any furniture easily out of the way as needed to follow along with an exercise video.

345 Treat Yourself to Proper Equipment

Exercising at home saves you the cost of a gym membership. Take some of the money that you have saved and invest in good-quality equipment. There are various options, including free weights, rowing machines, and treadmills.

Get Better Sleep

Research suggests that the quality of your sleep can have an effect on your IBS symptoms. You may have noticed that your symptoms are worse after a bad night's sleep. Luckily, there are some things that you can do to help you sleep soundly through the night.

346 Put Yourself on a Schedule

Our bodies have internal clocks that are regulated by the body's natural biorhythms. You can help your body to strengthen these rhythms by going to bed and waking up on a regular schedule that you stick to closely. This may mean no more sleeping in on the weekends!

347 Don't Drink Caffeine Late in the Day

You certainly wouldn't give a baby a cup of coffee before bedtime. Caffeine is a stimulant, so any late-day consumption puts you at risk for tossing and turning. Don't drink anything containing caffeine for at least eight hours before bed.

348 Keep Your Alcohol Intake to a Minimum

It is a well-established fact that too much alcohol can disturb the quality of your sleep. More than one or two drinks per day is enough to significantly impair your ability to sleep deeply.

349 Avoid Eating a Heavy Meal before Bedtime

Sleep is the time for your body to rest. It can't rest if it is still digesting your last meal. Eat your dinner several hours before bedtime and keep your late-night snacking light.

350 Don't Exercise Too Close to Bedtime

Regular exercise is actually very good for your sleep habits—as long as it is not too late in the evening. Try to complete your workout at least three hours before bed.

351 Take Your Shower at Night

Most parents learn early on that giving their child a warm bath in the evenings makes for a smoother bedtime transition. There is actually a physiological reason for this: a cooling body induces drowsiness. So, if you are not at too much risk for ruining your hairstyle, think about showering at night rather than in the morning.

352 Practice Those Relaxation Exercises Late in the Evening

A relaxed body is going to sleep better. Therefore, the late evening is a great time to practice your visualization, deep breathing, and muscle relaxation skills. Just make sure you practice in a comfortable chair so that you are training your body to relax, not to fall asleep. Once you are feeling more relaxed, you can transfer into your comfy bed.

353 Avoid Electronics for an Hour before Bed

There is some preliminary research indicating that the light emitted from electronic devices can impair your sleep. Even if that turns out not to be the case, electronics can be very stimulating to the brain. Watching TV or reading a book for the last hour of your day is more likely to promote sleepiness. So check your smartphone and Facebook one last time, then put your devices away, and snuggle in for your evening.

354 Don't Sleep with the TV On

Many people like to fall asleep with the television on. The problem with this is that part of getting a good night's sleep is the ability to fall back asleep if you are awakened. This is harder to do if you need the TV to fall asleep. Therefore, it would be best to try to wean yourself off TV as a sleep aid and turn the set off at your scheduled lights-out time.

355 Don't Look at the Clock!

Just as you would do with a child, tell yourself that *lights out* means lights out. Likewise, you wouldn't go into your child's room and announce the time loudly every hour or two. But if you obsessively look at the time when you are lying in bed, you are doing just that! You can turn the clock away from you to avoid worrying about the fact that you are awake and that you will feel lousy the next day (more on this in Tip 358!).

356 Write Down Your Worries, Then Put Them Out of Your Mind

If your brain tends to race with anxious thoughts when you are lying in bed, it can be quite helpful to keep a small notebook on your nightstand. There you can quickly jot down the things that are on your mind and then put the notebook away. Remind yourself that it is time to sleep. Problem solving can wait until the sun comes up.

357 Tell Yourself a Bedtime Story

Some busy minds have difficulty quieting down. Although counting sheep may have worked in a simpler past, this strategy is not quite as effective today given the pace of modern life. It can be helpful to give your brain a job. Think about a peaceful or enjoyable memory and relive the whole experience. Imagine a great vacation or a walk through your favorite city or forest.

358 Enjoy the Rest

Sleep studies show that people actually get more sleep than they think they do. We don't really have control over how much sleep we get, but we do have control over how much rest we get. So rather than fretting if you find that you are not sleeping, focus on the fact that you are warm and comfortable in your nice bed. Enjoy the fact that you now have time to enjoy that bedtime story you are relating to yourself. Keeping yourself calm will help soothe you back to sleep.

Beyond IBS

359 Your Body Can't Be Well Unless You Are Living a Well-Rounded Life

Health doesn't come about just because of a healthy diet or finding just the right combination of medications. Health comes from living a meaningful, satisfying life. Although your IBS may limit the activities you can pursue, it is important to find ways to ensure that your life isn't just about your illness.

360 Take Time for Play

Play doesn't have to mean structured athletics (although that's fine if you love it and your body cooperates). It simply means taking breaks from responsibility. Interact with a pet, get silly with your kids, or play a game on your mobile device.

361 Find Creative Outlets

Another way to avoid feeling defined or confined by your IBS is to spend time being creative. Try to remember what you liked doing as a kid, before concerns about performance took some of the joy out of things. Did you like to paint, draw, or write poems? Cooking can be a very creative outlet and will certainly help you in preparing healthy meals that sit well with your body. Schedule some time each week to do whatever it is that gets your creative juices flowing.

362 Whenever Possible, Avoid Toxic Relationships or Situations

It is hard to be healthy if you frequently find yourself in situations where you are being abused, whether that be physically or mentally. Certainly it is not always so easy to extricate yourself from an abusive relationship or a stressful job, but it is important to remember that you don't deserve to be abused. If you can pull away from a stressful situation, give yourself permission to do so. If not, seek therapy or use stress management techniques to help offset the effects of such toxicity on your health.

363 Find Meaningful Work

It is part of the human condition to want to add value to the world. Even if you don't like your job, look for some sense of pride or meaning in your labor. Another option is to engage in some sort of volunteer work—work that feeds your soul.

364 Learn a New Skill

It is good for your brain to spend some time learning something different. Whether that involves going back to school for additional formal education or simply taking a knitting class through adult education, look for opportunities to work and challenge your brain.

365 Nurture Your Spiritual Side

We are more than our bodies and our busy minds. Whatever your religious beliefs may be, research has shown that people with strong spiritual beliefs tend to be healthier and have a better response to medical care than those without such a foundation. You can nurture your spiritual side through formal religion if that is what works for you or through something as simple as spending time with Mother Nature. The point is to get in touch with the notion that we are all connected to something bigger than ourselves, something that transcends today's challenges.

Essential Resources

Helpful Websites

Irritable Bowel Syndrome at About.com
http://ibs.about.com
Articles written by Barbara B. Bolen, PhD, about all aspects of IBS, including symptoms, diagnosis, treatment, diet, and coping.

Irritable Bowel Syndrome Self Help and Support Group
www.ibsgroup.org
This site hosts the largest online IBS forum. Information is available on every aspect of dealing with IBS.

International Foundation for Functional Gastrointestinal Disorders
www.iffgd.org
This site is a resource for reliable medical information regarding IBS and offers a Care Locator service to help connect you with qualified professionals. In addition, the IFFGD is heavily involved in advocacy efforts for people who have functional gastrointestinal disorders like IBS.

Everything Low-FODMAP
www.everythinglowfodmap.com
This site, hosted by Barbara B. Bolen, PhD, and Kathleen Bradley, CPC, offers low-FODMAP training, recipes, and diet updates.

IBS Impact
www.ibsimpact.com
This site reflects the work of a grassroots advocacy effort for people with IBS.

IBS Network
www.theibsnetwork.org
This UK-based organization offers information and support for those who have IBS as well as for professionals who work with IBS patients.

Best Mobile Apps

The Monash University Low FODMAP Diet App

This app is a must-have for anyone following the low-FODMAP diet. It offers up-to-date information on the FODMAP content of a wide variety of foods. The app allows you to quickly search a food to see if it is high or low in FODMAPs.

The SoundsLikeIBS App

This app was developed by Michael Mahoney, author of the widely popular IBS Audio Program 100™. It provides you with access to the full hypnotherapy program through your mobile device.

Favorite Books

The Everything® Guide to the Low-FODMAP Diet: A Healthy Plan for Managing IBS and Other Digestive Disorders, by Barbara B. Bolen, PhD, and Kathleen Bradley, CPC
This comprehensive guide presents the science behind the diet, step-by-step instructions for following the diet, and includes 150 low-FODMAP, gluten-free recipes.

Breaking the Bonds of Irritable Bowel Syndrome: A Psychological Approach to Regaining Control of Your Life, by Barbara B. Bolen, PhD
This book offers a comprehensive cognitive behavioral therapy (CBT) self-help approach for managing IBS symptoms.

The First Year: IBS (Irritable Bowel Syndrome)—An Essential Guide for the Newly Diagnosed, by Heather Van Vorous
This book, written by a person who has IBS, provides you with wonderful tips for living with IBS.

A New IBS Solution: Bacteria—The Missing Link in Treating Irritable Bowel Syndrome, by Mark Pimentel, MD
This book provides information regarding the role of small intestinal bacteria overgrowth (SIBO) in IBS.

The Inside Tract: Your Guide to Great Digestive Health, by Gerard E. Mullin, MD, and Kathie Madonna Swift, MS, RD, LDN
This book offers a comprehensive discussion of your digestive system with dietary-based treatment plans for digestive disorders.

Bibliography

Bohm, M., Siwiec, R. M., & Wo, J. M. (2013). Diagnosis and management of small intestinal bacterial overgrowth. *Nutrition in Clinical Practice, 28,* 289–299.

Cash, B. D., Schoenfeld, P., & Chey, W. D. (2002). The utility of diagnostic tests in irritable bowel syndrome patients: A systematic review. *American Journal of Gastroenterology, 97,* 2812–2819.

Ford, A. C., (2014). American College of Gastroenterology monograph on the management of irritable bowel syndrome and chronic idiopathic constipation. *American Journal of Gastroenterology, 109,* S2–S26.

Gerson, M-J., Gerson, C. D., Awad, R. A., Dancey, C., Poitras, P., Porcelli, P., & Sperber, A. D. (2006). An international study of irritable bowel syndrome: Family relationships and mind-body attributions. *Social Science & Medicine, 62,* 2838–2847.

Gibson, P. R., & Shepherd, S. J. (2010). Evidence-based dietary management of functional gastrointestinal symptoms: The FODMAP approach. *Journal of Gastroenterology & Hepatology, 25,* 252–258.

Minocha, A., & Ademec, C. (2011). *The digestive system and digestive disorders* (2nd ed.). New York, NY: Facts on File.

Shepherd, S. J., & Gibson, P. (2013). *The Complete Low-FODMAP Diet.* New York, NY: The Experiment.

Acknowledgments

This book was the brainchild of Julia Pastore from Demos Health. Her enthusiasm for the project was infectious and her editing was first-class. Working with her has been an absolute pleasure.

I would also like to thank the powers that be at About.com who have given me the tremendous opportunity and responsibility to be the About.com IBS Expert. It is truly awe-inspiring that I have the ability to improve the lives and health of people around the globe through my words.

I would also like to thank my cowriters at About.com. They are a group of the most intelligent, talented, and make-you-laugh-out-loud funny people that I have ever met. I am so thankful to them for keeping me entertained during my workday and for inspiring me to always put out the best work that I can.

Last, I would like to thank my family for loving me and supporting me in all the wild and wacky directions that my career has taken me. I am truly blessed.

Index

meals *(cont.)*
  eating slowly, 56
  light, 54
  to lose weight, 46–48
  packing own, 90–91
  regular, 55
  size of, 42
  skipping, 42, 54
meats, 9, 47
medical care, 19–26. *See also* doctors
  diagnostic tests, 16, 21–22
  emergency, 24–26
  treatment options, 22–24
medications
  antibiotics, 24, 133
  antidepressants, 23
  antispasmodics, 23
  gut-directed, 24
  options for, 22–24
  over-the-counter (OTC), 16, 32–37
  questions about, 16
  side effects, 16
  Solesta, 24
  while traveling, 92
meditation, 30–31, 120, 127
methylcellulose, 35
microflora, 54, 133
milk of magnesia, 35
mind–body treatments, 29–31, 73
mindfulness, 30–31, 85, 122, 126–127
Miralax, 35
Monash University low-FODMAP
    diet app, 66
money worries, 128–129
motility problems, 5, 42
muscle tension, 120

Nature, 121, 142
non-celiac gluten sensitivity (NCGS), 7
nuts, 9

oligosaccharides, 66
omega-3 fatty acids, 41, 53
online support groups, 96

organic produce, 43
osmotic laxatives, 35
outdoors, 121
overeating, 42
over-the-counter (OTC) medications,
    32–37
  for constipation, 33–35
  for diarrhea, 36
  for gas and bloating,
    36–37
  questions about, 16
  while traveling, 92

pain
  abdominal, 5, 7, 73
  management, 73, 112
  severity of, 14
pain scale, 14
Paleo diet, 70
parenting, 111–112
peppermint oil, 32–33
peppermint tea, 44, 81
pesticides, 43
physical exercise, 48, 81, 91,
    134–137, 138–139
physical therapy, 32
physicians. *See* doctors
play, 141
polyols, 66–67
portable toilets, 80, 92
portion sizes, 42
positive thinking,
    121–124
prebiotics, 43, 68
primary care doctor, 13
probiotics, 43, 133–134
probiotic supplements, 36–37,
    133–134
processed foods
  avoiding, 134
  gluten-free, 63
procrastination habits, 86
productivity, 125
progressive muscle relaxation
    (PMR), 120

About the Author

Dr. Barbara Bolen is a psychologist, health coach, and health writer specializing in digestive health. In addition to running a private psychotherapy practice and health coaching business, she currently serves as the IBS Expert for the website About.com. She is author of *Breaking the Bonds of Irritable Bowel Syndrome* and co-author of *The Everything® Guide to the Low-FODMAP Diet* and *IBS Chat: Real Life Stories and Solutions*. She is also the co-creator of the Low-FODMAP Diet Training Program™ and the Low-FODMAP Diet E-Course™. Dr. Bolen's education and experience in psychology, medical research, and nutrition provide her with a unique background for helping people to optimize their mental, digestive and overall health.

drbarbarabolen.com

Printed in the United States
By Bookmasters